Renal Diet Cookbook

A Comprehensive Guide to Manage Kidney Disease, Avoid Dialysis and Improve your Health. Tasty Recipes with Low Sodium, Potassium and Phosphorus

Eva Moore

© Copyright 2019 by Eva Moore
All rights reserved.

This document is geared towards providing exact and reliable information with regard to the topic and issue covered. The publication is sold with the idea that the publisher is not required to render accounting, officially permitted or otherwise qualified services. If advice is necessary, legal or professional, a practiced individual in the profession should be ordered.

- From a Declaration of Principles which was accepted and approved equally by a Committee of the American Bar Association and a Committee of Publishers and Associations.

In no way is it legal to reproduce, duplicate, or transmit any part of this document in either electronic means or printed format. Recording of this publication is strictly prohibited, and any storage of this document is not allowed unless with written permission from the publisher. All rights reserved.

The information provided herein is stated to be truthful and consistent, in that any liability, in terms of inattention or otherwise, by any usage or abuse of any policies, processes, or directions contained within is the sole and utter responsibility of the recipient reader. Under no circumstances will any legal responsibility or blame be held against the publisher for any reparation, damages, or monetary loss due to the information herein, either directly or indirectly.

Respective authors own all copyrights not held by the publisher.

The information herein is offered for informational purposes solely and is universal as so. The presentation of the information is without contract or any type of guarantee assurance.
The trademarks that are used are without any consent, and the publication of the trademark is without permission or backing by the trademark owner. All trademarks and brands within this book are for clarifying purposes only and are the owned by the owners themselves, not affiliated with this document

TABLE OF CONTENTS

ABOUT THE BOOK ....

INTRODUCTION ....

CHAPTER I: AN OVERVIEW AND STUDY ON KIDNEY DISEASE 1

    Definition 1

    Causes of kidney disease 1

    Symptoms of kidney disease 2

    Stages of kidney disease 3

CHAPTER II: EFFECTIVELY MANAGING KIDNEY DISEASE 4

    Control your blood pressure 4

    Engage in physical activities 5

    Stop smoking 6

    Get enough rest 8

    Engage in healthy ways to manage stress level: the most effective method to oversee and diminish pressure 9

CHAPTER III: RENAL DIET 13

    Sodium 13

    What Is Sodium and Its Job In The Body? 13

    For what reason should kidney patients examine sodium consumption? 14

    By what method would patients be able to check/gauge their sodium consumption? 14

    Potassium 15

What Is Potassium and Its Job In The Body? 15

In What Manner Would Patients Be Able to Screen Their Potassium Consumption? 15

Phosphorus 16

What is Phosphorus and its job in the body? 16

By what method would patients be able to screen their Phosphorus admission? 16

Protein 17

Liquids 17

Food Combination Fitting for Breakfast 17

Food Combinations Fitting For Lunch 21

Chocolate in renal diet 23

More Lunch and Packed Lunch Renal diet Ideas 23

Snacks, Soups and Starters 25

Vegetarian Dishes 28

The Versatile Mince Section - for vegetarians too 31

Simple Chicken Dishes 37

Simple Meat Dishes 41

Fish Dishes 44

Side Dishes 49

Puddings and Cakes 52

Christmas Recipes 58

Main renal diet dishes (full dish) with nutritional benefits 65

Combination meals 78

CHAPTER IV: FOOD TO AVOID FOR A HEALTHY KIDNEY........ 97

1. Dark-Colored Colas 98

2. Avocados 99

3. Canned Foods 99

4. Whole-Wheat Bread 100

5. Brown Rice 100

6. Bananas 101

7. Dairy 101

8. Oranges and Orange Juice 102

9. Processed Meats 102

10. Pickles, Olives, and Relish 103

11. Apricots 103

12. Potatoes 104

13. Soda 104

14. Butter 105

15. Mayonnaise 105

16. Frozen foods 105

17. Tomatoes 106

18. Swiss Chard, Spinach and Beet Greens 106

19. Dates, Raisins, and Prunes 106

20. Pretzels, Chips, and Crackers 107

EXTRA TIP 107

CHAPTER V: ACHIEVING WEIGHT LOSS WITH RENAL DIET..108

Why some people on Renal want to lose weight?..108

Weight-loss guide for individuals on renal diet 108

Weight-loss diet guide for individuals on renal diet..................................109

Exercise with your doctor's consent 109

Portion size consideration..109

Self-Appreciation..110

Hindrances when carrying out weight-loss routines..................................110

Physical: Anemia...110

    Post-treatment..110

    Peritoneal dialysis (PD) 111

    Adequate protein 111

Emotional: Food choices 111

    Keeping the course..111

SUMMARY 113

CONCLUSION..114

How to be successful in the renal diet program...114

About the book

A comprehensive guide to manage kidney disease, avoid dialysis, and improve your health, is a book aimed at aiding persons who want to improve their general health with the correct diets and knowledge related kidney disease.

Introduction

Health is wealth as it is generally accepted, but I beg to add and say only good health can equal wealth. For good health become a reality, a proper diet is very much-needed, as this diet is a very crucial part of managing kidney disease and improve your overall health.

Kidney disease though chronic, but it isn't an automatic death sentence, with the right guide, diet, and checkup, one can live a healthy life as though no disease was ever in view.

It is right that before providing a solution to a question, the question itself should be reviewed and understood. So, in the first few chapters of this incredible diet book, the subject kidney disease, its causes, effects, stages would be discussed, which would lead us to renal diet and how to improve our health with its special procedures.

CHAPTER I: An overview and study on kidney disease

Definition

In a state whereby the kidney can no longer perform its primary functions, it can be said that a person suffers from kidney disease or impairment of the kidney. The Kidney works on effectively to getting rid of waste/unnecessary materials present in the body, which is gotten from the food you consume. The kidneys are responsible for the excretion of urea which is a dietary protein, sodium, phosphate, and potassium. If the kidney is damaged or compromised, then these materials build up and thus become harmful to your body and health in general. The kidney has various vital functions, which include:
- the management of pH level and of ion quantities,
- removal of waste and administration of osmolarity,
- regulation of ion concentrations,
- production of hormones, as well as the management of extracellular fluid volume.

The kidneys ensure to support the required amount of plasma to keep the blood flow sufficient to the vital organs.

Causes of kidney disease

The most common causes of End-stage renal disease (Kidney Failure) are HBP (High blood pressure) and Diabetes. Other possible causes include: Autoimmune diseases such as lupus and Urinary tract infections as well as genetic disorders such as polycystic kidney disease (it is hereditary), Nephrotic syndrome etc.

Acute renal failure (ARF) is a case whereby the kidney suddenly stops working. Common causes of acute renal failure include heart attack, insufficient flow of blood to the kidney, urinary tract infections and illegal drug use and drug abuse.

ARF is a form of kidney failure which is mostly temporary. Your kidney functions may return to normal with the appropriate treatment and if there is no trace of other major health complications.

Symptoms of kidney disease

We would look at some signs of kidney disease. Indeed, all symptoms may not be clear at once; below are some that are dominant.
1. Reduced appetite: this is a general symptom, which can be caused by reduced kidney function resulting from the build-up of toxins.

2. Swelling on the ankle and feet: when there is high sodium retention, caused by a reduction in kidney function, which leads to swelling in feet and ankle. This aforementioned sign can also be an indication of heart disease or liver disease.

3. Experiencing trouble sleeping: at the point where the kidney is damaged, and it fails to filter waste products effectively, the toxins remain in the blood, thereby making sleeping difficult.

4. Tiredness, lack of concentration, and low energy: anemia, which is a state whereby little oxygen gets to the brain, is related to kidney failure. This will lead to loss of concentration, and also loss of memory.

5. Foul taste of food: when there is an inadequate removal of toxins, there is a build-up of waste, this waste is referred to as uremia. When this is present, food begins to taste like metal, and it also causes bad breath, loss of appetite, and eventually loss of weight.

6. Severe itching: as mentioned above, the kidney helps to remove toxins from the blood, but when this does not work, it also leads to severe itching, which, if not carefully addressed, leads to deformation of the skin layers.

7. Cramping of muscles: low phosphorus or low calcium level may lead to muscle cramping.

8. The coloration of urine: Kidneys produce urine. When there is kidney failure, you may experience changes in urine color due to mixture with blood and other toxins.

Stages of kidney disease

The various stages of kidney disease are solely dependant on kidney functions and the resulting damage.

1. Stage one: At this stage, the kidney damage is low, and there are still normal kidney functions. The GFR (glomerular filtration rate) is ≥ 90 ml/min/1.73 m2

2. Stage two: In this stage, there is a mild loss of kidney functions. The GFR is 60-89 ml/min/1.73 m2

3. Stage three: In this stage, there is a noticeable loss of kidney functions. This stage is in two grades, namely, stage three and stage three b. The GFR is 45-59 ml/min/1.73 m2 and 30-44 ml/min/1.73 m2, respectively.

4. Stage four: In this stage, there is severe loss of kidney functions. The GFR is 15-29 ml/min/1.73 m2

5. Stage five: This stage is referred to as End-stage renal disease. In this stage, there is Kidney failure and the need for transplant or dialysis. The GFR is less than 15 ml/min/1.73 m2

CHAPTER II: Effectively Managing Kidney Disease

Kidney disease is in no way an automatic death sentence, as it can be managed with the right knowledge. People with kidney disease, whatever the stage may be, can live a healthy life. Below and some steps that can be used to improve the living of a CKD patient qualitatively.

Control your blood pressure

If by chance you have hypertension, your health care supplier has to be aware, and you both need to cooperate as a group to diminish it. You two need to concur on your BP goal. Together, you should think of an arrangement and timetable for arriving at your aim. BP (blood pressure) is typically estimated in mmHg. Contact your doctor to get help in the primary approach to the disease: detect blood pressure and pulse level. Checking your blood strain at home between visits to your PCP can be helpful. You likewise might need to carry a relative with you when you visit your doctor. Having a loved one who is aware of your hypertension and who comprehends what you have to do to bring down your pulse frequently, makes it simpler to roll out the improvements that will aid you with arriving at your goal. The steps recorded in this book will help bring down your circulatory strain. In the event that you have ordinary blood strain or prehypertension, following these means will help keep you from growing hypertension and to have a good control of your blood pressure. This book is intended to help you with embracing a more advantageous way of life and make sure to take recommended blood strain reducing medications. Following the guide outlined will assist you with averting and control hypertension. While you read them, ponder internally . . ."I Can accomplish this!"

Engage in physical activities

Type of Exercise

Pick constant action, such as, strolling, swimming, bicycling (inside or out), skiing, vigorous moving, or some other exercises where you have to move substantial muscle bunches consistently. Low-level fortifying activities may likewise be a vital part of your program which will turn out to be helpful. Structure your plan to utilize low loads and high redundancies, and stay away from hard work.

To What Extent to Exercise

Work toward 30 minutes a session. You should develop progressively to this level. There is nothing supernatural around 30 minutes. If you want to walk 45 to an hour, go ahead. Make sure to pursue the guidance recorded under "When should I quit working out?" in this pamphlet.

How Often to Exercise

Exercise at any rate for at least 3-days per week. This ought to be non-back to back days, for instance, Monday, Wednesday, and Friday. Three days a week, is the base prerequisite to accomplish the advantages of your activity.

How Hard to Work While Exercising?

This is the hardest to discuss without knowing your very own activity limit. This is the most difficult to discuss without knowing the activity limit. For example, if you have breathing difficulties, you should not limit yourself in your motor activity. (It is useful not to practice a sport alone, if it is the first approach). During training, you should feel good and normal within an hour after training. Otherwise, if you feel uncomfortable in an hour, then slow down next time.

So much muscle irritation, should not be felt to a point where it shields you from practicing the following session. The power ought to be on an "agreeable push" level.

Begin gradually every session to heat up; get your pace, and then delayed down again when you are going to wrap up. The Most significant thing is to begin gradually and proceed progressively, enabling your body to adjust to the expanded degrees of action.

When Would It Be Advisable for Me to Work Out?
Try to schedule your activity into your typical day. Here are a few thoughts about when to work out: when you've eaten a huge dinner, wait at least one hour before training. If it's during the day, try to keep away from the hot weather (its best to work out during the cool part of the day). Morning or night is by all accounts the most ideal hours for working out. And to add lastly, try not to work out when its less than an hour before bedtime.

When Would It Be Advisable for Me To Quit Working Out?
Everything must be done with caution, exercise inclusive. If by feel extremely weak and tired during or before work out, it is advisable to quit, if they are discomforting pains in the chest, fast heartbeats, spasms in your leg or thighs, or you are feeling woozy or dazed. All these are signs that say "Hey! You got to take a break," and you better do.

Are There Any Occasions When I Ought Not to Work Out?
Indeed, you ought not to practice without having a conversation with your doctor if any of the following happens before your work out time: if you have changed your dialysis plan, you have changed your prescription timetable, if you are running temperature, your physical condition has changed, you have eaten excessively, or you have bone issues that become more terrible with work out.

Stop smoking

What is the link between smoking and kidney functionality?
Smoking is an easy one-way ticket for Renal failure. People who smoke, have a high rate of chance to develop renal failure when in comparison with non-smokers.

Smoking expands pulse, circulatory strain, blood clump arrangement, and advances fat stores in the supply routes. These are, all probability, smoking-related procedures that can prompt renal capacity being influenced.

Compared with non-smokers, smokers have an expanded danger of the following, protein in pee, diabetic-related kidney harm and practically twofold the pace of movement to end-organize Renal Failure, twice prone to create kidney disease compared with non-smokers (the more prominent the measure of cigarettes every day smoked, the more serious the danger of creating kidney disease).

What Are the Medical Advantages for Renal Diet Patients Who Quit Smoking?
Quitting smoking not simply lessens the threat of creating various diseases, it may help a patient recover quicker by discarding the extraordinary effects of tobacco on the body. It might help kidney moderate workload decline in people with type two diabetes and kidney disease. It helps in slowing the development of kidney infections in people with diabetes who use drugs called ACE inhibitors. Additionally, helps to lessen the threat of kidney infections and to reduce the peril of smoking-related progression and development of various sorts of neuropathy (damage to the peripheral sensory system).

In the Wake of Stopping Smoking
Your wellbeing will start to improve after only 20 minutes, and you will before long begin to see the advantages of stopping.

After 20 minutes, your circulatory strain and heartbeat rate will have returned to the average pace of a non-smoker.

After 24 hours, carbon monoxide will be gone from your body. Your lungs will begin to get out undesirable bodily fluid and smoking flotsam and jetsam.

After 48 hours, nourishment will begin to taste better, and your feeling of smell will improve as well.

After 72 hours, your breathing will become more straightforward, and your vitality levels will increment.

After 2-12 weeks, your flow will improve, making your skin look better.

After 3-9 months, smoker's hacks and breathing issues ought to improve as your lung work increments by up to 10%.

After five years, your danger of a coronary episode will tumble to about a large portion of that of a smoker.

After ten years, your danger of malignant lung growth will tumble in no small portion of that of smoke, and your risk of a respiratory failure should be equivalent to somebody who has never smoked.

Get enough rest

A decent night's rest is critical to your general prosperity and, it turns out, your kidneys.

Scientists have just connected the effect of poor sleeping habits and rest issue to higher likelihood of diabetes and cardiovascular sickness. Now the connection between shut-eye and kidney work is turning out to be more transparent with new research by leading scientists.

Kidney work is really directed by the rest wake cycle. It helps organize the kidneys' outstanding task at hand for more than 24 hours.

Examinations carried out by leading scientists, will investigate melatonin emission, which is the hormone our bodies produce normally to sync our nighttime capacities. As a feature of the examination, sound members will have their rest confined, and their hormone levels and kidney capacity will be estimated.

The examination will likewise incorporate individuals who are regularly rest confined and will request that they sleep longer hours to check whether it influences their physiology, circulatory strain, blood glucose levels, and kidney work. Half of this gathering will likewise be given melatonin enhancements to check whether that affects their kidney work after some time.

Better seeing how the kidneys function and to collaborate with our hormones around evening time may likewise help decide better sustenance rules and improved times for medicine conveyance. This is because the kidneys' capacity to process drugs and supplements like sodium and potassium changes among day and night.

The investigation could distinguish new gatherings of people who are at higher hazard for creating constant kidney disease because of their way of life or work routine, for instance, the individuals who work in shifts and those with interminable lack of sleep issues.

Engage in healthy ways to manage stress level: the most effective method to oversee and diminish pressure

Here, we might want to begin, by giving you a prologue to what stress is, the thing that indications of stress are, what practical guide you can carry out when feeling stressed and provide a pragmatic counsel to averting it, to show why we are energetic about moving towards a less focused on the country.

What is pressure?
Stress is an inclination of being under an abnormal weight. This weight or burden can be generated from different parts of your everyday life. For example, an expanded remaining burden, a transitional period, a contention you have with your family, or new and existing money related stresses. You may find that it has an aggregate impact, with every stressor expanding over each other.

During these circumstances, you may feel compromised or upset, and your body may make a pressure reaction. This can cause an assortment of physical side effects; change how you carry on and lead you to encounter progressively dangerous emotions.

Stress influences us in various manners, both physically and genuinely, and in differing intensities.

How Might I Distinguish the Indications of Stress?
Everybody encounters pressure. In any case, when it is influencing

your life, wellbeing, and prosperity, it is critical to handle it as quickly as time permits. Keeping in mind that pressure affects everybody unexpectedly, there are regular signs and side effects you can watch out for, which include the following: sentiments of consistent stress or tension, sentiments of being overpowered, trouble concentrating, state of mind swings or changes in your disposition, peevishness or having a touchiness, trouble unwinding, despondency, low confidence, eating pretty much than expected, utilizing liquor, tobacco or unlawful medications to unwind, a throbbing painfulness, especially muscle strain, looseness of the bowels and obstruction, sentiments of queasiness or coziness or/and loss of sex drive.

Just if you are encountering these indications for a drawn-out period, and feel they are influencing your regular day to day existence or are making you feel unwell, you ought to address your GP. You can request data about the help administrations and medicines accessible to you.

Three Stages to Take When Feeling Pushed
1. *Acknowledge when it is causing you an issue*
Attempt to make the association between feeling drained or sick and the weights you are looked at yourself.
Pay personal care to physical warnings, such as, tense muscles, over-tiredness, cerebral pains, or migraines.

2. *Recognize the causes*
Attempt to distinguish the fundamental causes
Sort the potential purposes behind your worry into three classifications:
I) those with a handy arrangement
II) those that will show signs of improvement given time and
III) those you can't take care of
Attempt to discharge the stress of those in the second and third gatherings and let them go

3. *Audit your way of life*
Can you be able to take on something over the top?
Are there things you are doing which could be given over to another person?

Would you be able to get things done in an all the easier way?

To follow up on the response to these inquiries, you may need to organize things you are trying to do and reorder your life.

This will discharge pressure that can emerge out of attempting to do everything simultaneously.

Seven Stages to Help Shield Yourself from Stress

1. Eat Healthily

Eating Healthy can diminish the dangers of diet-related diseases.

There is a developing measure of proof demonstrating how nourishment influences our moods and how eating actively can improve this.

You can secure your sentiments of prosperity by guaranteeing that your eating routine gives satisfactory measures of cerebrum supplements, for example, essential vitamins and minerals, just as water.

2. Know about smoking and drinking liquor

Do whatever it takes not to, or lessen the sum you smoke and drink liquor.

Although they may appear to lessen strain at first, this is deluding as they regularly make issues worse.

3. Exercise

Attempt to incorporate physical exercise into your way of life as it very well may be influential in soothing pressure.

Indeed, even only going out and getting some outside air, and taking some light physical exercise, such as taking a stroll to the shops can truly help.

4. Take break

Set aside some effort to unwind.

Find some harmony between an obligation to other people and duty to yourself; this can genuinely diminish feelings of anxiety.

Disclose to yourself that it is all right to organize self-care. Do you require break yet saying 'I can't take the downtime'? If so, read progressively about how taking a break is significant for good emotional well-being.

5. Be careful

Care is a mind-body way to deal with life that causes us to relate contrastively to encounters. It includes focusing on our contemplations and emotions such that expands our capacity to oversee troublesome circumstances and settle on savvy decisions.

Attempt to rehearse care normally

Care contemplation can be drilled anyplace.

Research has recommended that it can lessen the impacts of pressure, nervousness and related issues, such as sleep deprivation, poor fixation and low states of mind, in some people.

6. Get some relaxing rest

Is it safe to say that you are discovering you are battling to rest? This is a typical issue when you're stressed.

Could your physical or psychological wellness sway your capacity to rest?

Would you be able to alter your condition to help improve your rest?

Might you be able to get up as opposed to remaining in bed when your psyche is stressing around evening time?

Would you be able to roll out little improvements to your way of life to support you get a relaxing rest?

For full subtleties on tips on getting a decent night's rest read our guide How to rest better and ten top tips for good rest.

7. Try not to be excessively hard on yourself

Attempt to keep things in context.

Recall that having an awful day is a general human condition.

Just in case you stagger or feel you have fizzled, don't pound yourself.

Go about as though you were your very own closest companion: be benevolent and strong.

Take a couple of moments every day to appreciate yourself.

CHAPTER III: Renal diet

Individuals with compromised kidney work must hold fast to a renal or kidney diet to eliminate the measure of waste in their blood. Squanders in the blood originate from nourishment and fluids that are expended. At the point when kidney work is undermined, the kidneys, not channel or evacuate squander appropriately. In the situation that waste is left in the blood, it can adversely influence a patient's electrolyte levels. After a kidney diet may likewise help advance kidney work and moderate the movement of complete kidney failure.

A renal eating routine is one that low content level of phosphorus, protein and sodium. A renal eating regimen additionally underlines the significance of devouring high-quality protein and typically constraining liquids. A few patients may likewise need to restrain potassium and calcium. Each individual's body is extraordinary, and in this manner, it is pivotal that every patient works with a renal dietitian work to think of an eating regimen that is custom-fitted to the patient's needs.

The following are a few substances that are significant to check to advance a renal eating routine.

Sodium
What Is Sodium and Its Job In The Body?

This is a mineral that is mostly found in common nourishments. The vast majority consider salt and sodium as compatible. Salt, in any case, is a compound of both chloride and sodium. Nourishments we eat may contain salt, or they may contain sodium in different structures. Prepared nourishments regularly contain more significant levels of sodium because of included salt.

Sodium is one of the body's three significant electrolytes (potassium and chloride are the other two). Electrolytes control the liquids going all through the body's tissues and cells. Sodium adds to:
- Regulating pulse and blood volume;
- Regulating nerve capacity and muscle withdrawal;
- Regulating the corrosive base equalization of blood, and also balancing how much liquid the body keeps or dispenses with.

For what reason should kidney patients examine sodium consumption?

A high quantity levels of sodium can be unhealthy and unsafe for people who are suffering from any stage of kidney disease because their kidneys can't satisfactorily dispose of overabundance sodium and liquid from the body. As sodium and fluid develop in the tissues and circulatory system, they may cause:

1. Increased thirst

2. Edema: growing in the legs, hands, and face

3. High circulatory strain

4. Heart Failure: Too much liquid in your body system can exhaust your heart, making it expanded and feeble

5. Shortness of breath: liquid can develop in the lungs, making it hard to relax

By what method would patients be able to check/gauge their sodium consumption?

One can be able to check sodium consumptions by always reading nourishment marks.
- pay close attention to the size of food served;
- use fresh instead of packed meat;

- choose to consume no-salt included canned or solidified produce;
- compare brands and take things most minimal in sodium content;
- use flavors that don't include salt in their tags;
- cook at home rather than constantly eating out and ensure not to add salt;
- limit all out sodium substance to maximum of 400 milligrams for each supper and 150 milligrams for each bite.

Potassium
What Is Potassium and Its Job In The Body?

This is a mineral that is present in a considerable amount in various nourishments we eat and is additionally found generally in the body. Potassium assumes a job in keeping the heartbeat customary and the muscles working accurately. Potassium is likewise fundamental for keeping up liquid and electrolyte balance in the circulation system. The kidneys help to keep the required amount of potassium content in your body, and they remove abundance sums into the pee.

For what reason should kidney patients screen their potassium consumption?

When the kidneys come up short, they can never again eliminate the overabundance potassium, so its levels develop in the body. High level of potassium that is present in the blood is called hyperkalemia, which can cause muscle shortcoming, a sporadic heartbeat, slow beat, heart attacks, and ultimately Death.

In What Manner Would Patients Be Able to Screen Their Potassium Consumption?

At the point when the kidneys never again manage potassium, a patient must screen the measure of potassium that enters the body.

These are tips to help maintain the required level of potassium content in your body (Bloodstream). They include:
- trying to talk with a renal dietitian about making an eating arrangement;
- limit milk and dairy things to 8 oz consistently;
- choose fresh foods grown from the ground;

- limit nourishments that have high potassium content;
- read names on packaged nourishment and avoid potassium chloride;
- pay close regard for serving size and keep a nourishment journal.

Phosphorus
What is Phosphorus and its job in the body?
This type of mineral is essential in bone advancement and support. Phosphorus likewise aids the improvement of connective tissue and organs and helps in muscle development. When nourishment containing phosphorus is devoured and processed, the small digestion tracts ingest the phosphorus, so it tends to be put away during the bones.

For what reason should kidney patients screen Phosphorus consumption?
Normal working kidneys can remove extra phosphorus in your blood. Exactly when kidney work is undermined, the kidneys never again empty excess phosphorus. When there is high phosphorus content in the blood, it leads to the weakening of the bones due to the removal of calcium.

By what method would patients be able to screen their Phosphorus admission?
Phosphorus can be found in numerous nourishments. Accordingly, patients with compromised kidney capacity should work with a renal dietitian to help oversee phosphorus levels.

Tips to help protect phosphorus at levels
These are tips to help on protecting their phosphorus level:
- know what nourishments are lower in phosphorus;
- pay close regard for serving size;
- eat just a little of high protein-containing foods as supper and for snacks;
- eat new foods grown from the ground;
- ask your doctor about utilizing phosphate folios at feast time and keep a nourishment diary.

Protein

Protein isn't an issue for healthy kidneys. Ordinarily, protein is ingested, and squander items are made, which thus are sifted by the nephrons of the kidney. At that point, with the assistance of extrarenal proteins, the waste transforms into pee. Conversely, harmed kidneys neglect to evacuate protein waste, and it aggregates in the blood.

The best possible use of protein is precarious for Chronic Kidney Disease patients as the sum contrasts with each phase of the illness. Protein is essential for tissue upkeep and other real jobs, so it is necessary to eat the prescribed quantity for the particular stage of sickness, as indicated by your nephrologist or renal dietician.

Liquids

Liquid control is significant for patients in the later phases of Chronic Kidney Disease since ordinary liquid utilization may cause the liquid to develop in the body, which could get perilous. Individuals on dialysis frequently have diminished pee yield, so expanded liquid in the body can put unnecessary weight on the individual's heart and lungs.

A patient's liquid remittance is determined on an individual premise, contingent upon pee yield and dialysis settings. It is crucial to pursue your nephrologist's/nutritionist's fluid admission rules.

To control liquid admission, patients should not drink more than what your primary care physician orders, count all nourishments that will soften at room temperature, be mindful of the measure of liquids used in cooking.

Food Combination Fitting for Breakfast

Welcome to the breakfast section. The goal is to offer various meals, their benefits, and preparation technique that would suit your morning and help you avoid dialysis.

1. Fruit Salad and Yoghurt

This recipe uses tinned fruit instead of fresh fruit which is great if you are on a potassium constraint, reason being that tinned fruit is naturally lower in potassium. Just remember to drain out the juice off as this is where much of the potassium is.

Serves 1
- Tinned fruit, such as peaches, pears, or perhaps a fruit cocktail. Choose the ones tinned in juice if you are diabetic or are looking at losing weight. Otherwise, you can give the syrup model a trial.
- Yogurt of your choice. If you are looking at losing weight, ensure you go for the low fat yogurt or better still free fat yogurt. On the other hand, if you are struggling to keep your weight up, choose the full-fat yogurt or creamy yogurt.

Remember: if you are on a phosphate restriction then you should include the yogurt as a part of your ½ pint (300ml) milk allowance (e.g., a 125g yogurt is equal to125ml of milk).

2. The Bread Basket

Most plain bread is low in phosphate and potassium so here are some suggestions on the variety of plain bread available for breakfast. Try to pick the wholemeal varieties when this is possible. These bread can be served with: cream cheese, honey, jam, syrup, marmalade or an egg cooked to your taste.
- Ready-made shop-bought breakfast pancakes
- Crumpets (moderate in phosphates so have only occasionally)
- Brioche*
- English muffin
- Butter croissants*
- Plain bagel

*These items have high fat contents, so be cautious if you are looking at losing weight.

EXTRA: English Breakfast Traditionally Cooked

This particular breakfast is avoided by so many people due to its phosphate and potassium content that is quite high. However, by sticking to these guidelines, a cooked breakfast can very much be enjoyed occasionally.

Serves 1
- 1 egg – Whichever way you choose
- 2 pieces of bacon or 1 sausage (opt for low fat or free fat if you plan on losing weight)
- 4 small mushrooms or 2 tbsp of baked beans or 1 small tomato

- As much toast as you deem fit (although you should be careful if you plan on losing weight)

Preparation method
1. If you plan on losing weight, then grilling is the best cooking method or you can fry in a non stick frying pan with small quantity of oil or if spray oil is available that would work.
2. If you want to gain weight, then choose to fry in fat this will help increase the calories content of your breakfast.

3. High energy Porridge

This high energy recipe is useful if you are unintentionally losing weight or you are underweight. It contains extra calories which are needed.

Remember: if you are on phosphate or fluid restriction then the milk should be taken from your daily allowance for fluid and milk.

Serves 1
- 35g (1¼oz) porridge oats
- 200ml full-fat milk
- Optional: add cream and syrup or jam for extra energy

Preparation method
1. cook in the microwave for around 1-2 minutes, stirring at 30-second intervals.
2. Alternatively, mix all the ingredients in a pan, heat the pan, and boil for 3-4 min.

4. Healthy Porridge

In case you are quick to lose weight, this porridge can be the correct decision, it is low in calories and high in fiber, which will help you with feeling full for more, so you're less inclined to nibble before lunch. In the event that you are on a phosphate limitation you might need to attempt soy or rice milk to supplant the skimmed milk as this is lower in phosphate just as normally low fat.

Serves 1
- 35g (1¼oz) porridge oats

- 100ml skimmed milk
- 100ml water
- ½ grated apple
- Sprinkle of cinnamon

Preparation method
1. Mix all the ingredients in a pan, heat the pan, and boil for 3-4 min.
2. Alternatively cook in the microwave for around 1-2 minutes, stirring at 30-second intervals.

5. Homemade Granola

Many shop-bought granolas are unsuitable if you are after potassium and phosphate restrictions due to the high content of nuts and dried fruit. Here is an easy recipe to make your alternative oat breakfast, which can be served with milk, yogurt, or stewed fruits.

Tip smart: add dried cranberries as they are naturally lower in potassium than other dried fruit, but it will taste equally good without.

Makes up to 10 servings
- 4 tablespoons of sunflower or vegetable oil
- 2 tablespoons of clear honey or golden syrup
- 1 tablespoon of lemon juice
- 2 tablespoons of soft brown sugar
- 300g (10½oz) rolled oats
- Dried cranberries (optional)

Preparation method
1. Preheat the oven to 140°C (120°C Fan)/275°F/Gas
2. In a significant saucepan melt the oil, honey/syrup, lemon juice, and sugar over a low heat. The aim is not to let the mixture bubble, just to let the ingredients melt and mix. Then add the oats and stir well.
3. Spread the mixture out on a baking tray in an even layer (you may need two baking trays depending on the size of them. Bake in the oven for around 30-40 minutes until crisp. Check on the granola every 10 minutes and stir to ensure an even bake.
4. Once cooked and cooled you could add a few handfuls of dried

cranberries. The granola should be stored in an airtight container and it is used within one month.

Food Combinations Fitting For Lunch

Having a dietary restriction need not be over burdensome. This lunch section provides some kidney-friendly suggestions that you can have at home and away.

1. Rice, Pasta or Couscous Salad

Rice, pasta, and couscous are both low potassium alternatives to potato and make a filling alternative to bread. Try cold cooked rice, pasta or couscous mixed with tuna, ham or chicken and a range of vegetables such as sweet corn, cucumber, olives, peppers and some mayo. You could try flavouring it with some herbs or spices, for example dried basil, parsley, paprika, or even curry powder. A dash of salad dressing, a spoonful of pesto or stirring in soft white cream cheese can give it extra flavour.

2. Oatcake or Rice Cake Topping

Oat and rice cakes can be used as a healthy snack, and here are some suggestions for healthy toppings, which are also low in potassium and phosphate.
- Cottage cheese mixed with pineapple (canned and drained) or mixed with sweet corn (canned)
- Cottage cheese mixed with tuna, peas (pre-boiled or canned) and thyme
- Cream cheese mixed with garlic and chive or parsley, or any other herb or spice
- Lean ham topped with cream cheese
- Egg mayonnaise
- Tuna mayonnaise
- Tinned fish (without the bones as this makes them high in phosphate)

3.Sandwiches

Sandwiches could consist of bread, pitta, wraps, rolls or any other variety of bread available these days. The better option is always wholemeal as it contains more fiber but if you prefer white then opt for this occasionally. Here are some suggested fillings that provide

good sources of protein ideal for dialysis patients:
- Ham and cream cheese
- Chicken pesto and mayonnaise
- Tuna mayo with cucumber
- Coronation chicken (chicken mixed with mayonnaise and some curry powder)
- Cheese (within allowance), a small amount of salad and mayonnaise
- Egg and cress
- Sliced beef and horseradish or mustard
- Vegetarian sausage, chutney, and lettuce
- Sliced falafel with spring onions, chili sauce, and shredded lettuce
- Roasted red peppers, mozzarella, basil, and garlic mayonnaise
- Cream cheese and cucumber
- Turkey and cranberry sauce with lettuce
- Brie and cranberry
- Cheese (within allowance) and coleslaw

4. **Quiche**

Because it is made with eggs which are a good source of protein, quiche makes an excellent lunch to replace the protein lost during dialysis. Ready-made quiches are excellent but try to go for a low/reduced salt options (less than 1.5g per 100g). If you are trying to lose weight, then you might want to avoid the pastry and cook your quiche using the "pastry-less Quiche recipe" in the vegetarian section of this book.

EXTRA: Other Lunch Box Snacks
- Fruit such as apple, orange, pear (best option if you are trying to lose weight)
- Yogurt (within milk allowance if you're on a restriction) (try low fat or fat-free varieties if you are trying to lose weight)
- Mini packets of breadsticks
- Corn crisp, e.g. Skips, Dorritos, Monster Munch, Quavers, Wotsits, poppadoms, Tortilla chips (if you're trying to lose weight choose low calorie options, e.g. around 100kcal per packet). Crisps are naturally high in salt, so limit the number of times you enjoy these.
- Snackajacks, mini rice cakes, plain crackers, e.g. water biscuits
- Plain or butter popcorn (avoid the butter variety if you are trying

to lose weight)
- Prawn crackers
- Muffins
- Plain biscuits, e.g., Digestives, shortbread, Rich Tea
- Flapjacks (can be high in fat if you are trying to lose weight)
- Cereal bar (avoid any containing nuts or dried fruit)

Chocolate in renal diet

Chocolate is very high in potassium and phosphate regardless of whether its milk, white or dark chocolate, so if you are on a potassium or phosphate restriction, it is best to eat in moderation. If you decide to have some chocolate as an occasional treat, than opting for something that contains a small amount of chocolate is better than eating chunks of chocolate. For example, the foods all contain chocolate in small amounts:

- Small chocolate bar (wafer or biscuit based such as a Taxi, Kitkat or Penguin as they have less of the high phosphate chocolate).
- Chocolate digestives biscuits.
- Chocolate chip cookie (avoid double choc chip)
- Chocolate chip cereal bar
- Chocolate chip muffins or cake (again not double choc chip)

More Lunch and Packed Lunch Renal diet Ideas

1.   Goat's Cheese Rarebit

Don't be put off by the use of soya milk and goat's cheese in this recipe. They are both much lower in phosphate than cow's milk and cheddar and are equally tasty.

Serves 2-4
- 25g (¾oz) olive oil, vegetable spread or butter
- 150ml soya milk (used unsweetened one)
- 175g (6oz) soft goat's cheese
- 25g (¾oz) flour
- ½ tsp mustard
- pepper
- 2 egg yolks
- 4 slices bread

Preparation method
1. Place the spread or butter, soya milk, and cheese in a saucepan and heat gently until melted and smooth inconsistency.
2. Stir in the flour, and bring the mixture to the boil, stirring constantly while it thickens.
3. Remove from the heat and add the mustard and pepper. Leave to cool for 5 minutes, then whisk in the egg yolks with a fork.
4. Toast the bread on one side, turn over and divide the rarebit mixture between the slices.
5. Place under a hot grill and cook until bubbling and golden.

2.   Pesto Cream Veggie Dip

This dip recipe is great as a snack, a small meal, or as a dip to share with your guests. Using cream cheese makes it low in phosphate and if served with toasted pitta bread, crackers or corn crisps rather than potato crisps they would be low in potassium too.
- 200g (7oz) basil pesto
- 100g (3½oz) cream cheese
- 100g (3½oz) sour cream
- 2 tablespoons parmesan cheese

Preparation method
1. Place pesto, cream cheese, sour cream and Parmesan cheese in a bowl and stir well.
2. Mix until creamy and chill until ready to serve.

3. Smoked Mackerel Paté

Enjoy this low phosphate paté on toasted bread, Melba toast or any other crackers, if you are trying to lose weight then opt for the low-fat cream cheese.

Serves 1-6
- 200g (7oz) smoked mackerel fllets, skin removed
- 2 spring onions, trimmed and finely sliced
- 1 lemon
- 100g (3½oz) cream cheese
- 1 tablespoon creamed horseradish
- Pepper

Preparation method
1. Break the mackerel into chunks and finely chop it.
2. In a bowl add the mackerel, cream cheese, spring onions, creamed horseradish and zest of 1 lemon, then mix to combine.
3. Squeeze in the juice of your zested lemon, and mix again until you have a coarse paste.
4. Season to taste with pepper.

Snacks, Soups and Starters

Below are some very nice renal diet recipe for tasty soups that would keep you healthy.

1. Carrot and Coriander Soup

Carrots are a tasty low potassium vegetable, plus using a low salt stock means its kidney-friendly. Remember soup is fluid so count it if you're on a fluid restriction.

Serves 4
- 1 tbsp of vegetable or olive oil
- 1 onion, sliced
- 450g (1lb) carrots, sliced
- 1 tsp ground coriander
- 1.2 litres/2 pints vegetable stock such as low salt Bouillon
- 1 bay leaf
- Large bunch fresh coriander or fresh parsley, roughly chopped (optional)
- Freshly ground black pepper

Preparation method
1. Heat the oil in a large pan and add the onions and the carrots. Cook for 3-4 minutes until starting to soften.
2. Stir in the ground coriander and season well. Cook for 1 minute.
3. Add the vegetable stock and bay leaf and bring to the boil. Simmer until the vegetables are tender.
4. Remove the bay leaf and whizz the soup with a hand blender or in a blender until smooth. Reheat in a clean pan, stir in the fresh coriander or parsley and serve with some crusty bread.

2. Chicken Soup

Making homemade chicken soup is a great way to use up left-over roast chicken, vegetables, and stock. If you are fluid restricted you may wish to consider having less fluid at other times to ensure you don't exceed your restriction. For example, you could have egg on toast instead of cereal and milk for breakfast or have a couple of biscuits after a meal instead of custard with a pudding. In this recipe, we discard the water from the boiled vegetables before adding the stock – this helps to lower the potassium content of the vegetables.

Serves 4
- 1 tbsp of vegetable or olive oil
- 1 leek
- 3 medium carrots
- 2 medium potatoes, peeled
- 1-liter low salt chicken stock
- 1 tbsp cornflower (if required, see below)
- 300g (10½oz) leftover roast chicken, shredded and skin removed
- 3 tbsp Greek yogurt or double cream
- Squeeze of lemon juice

Preparation method
1. Roughly chop the leeks, carrots, and potatoes and boil in a large pot of water until tender.
2. Drain the vegetables and potatoes (do not reuse the cooking water), return to the pot, and add the stock.
3. Use a blender and blend the soup to your preferred consistency.
4. If you like soup to be thicker: return the pan to the hob on a low heat, mix the cornflower with a splash of cold water and add to the soup. Stir continuously while simmering until the soup thickens. Add the chicken and simmer for 5 minutes. To finish add the yogurt or cream and lemon juice.

3. Plain Scones

This is a staple recipe that works well as a small meal, snack or even a pudding and are low in both potassium and phosphate. Making 12 in one go might sound a lot but they freeze extremely well – just make sure you use them up within one month.

Makes 8-12
- 225g (8oz) self-raising flour
- pinch of salt
- 55g (2oz) butter
- 25g (1oz) caster sugar
- 150ml milk
- 1 free-range egg, beaten, to glaze (alternatively use a little milk)

Preparation method
1. Heat the oven to 220°C (200°C Fan)/425°F/Gas 7. Lightly grease a baking sheet.
2. Mix together the flour and salt and rub in the butter.
3. Stir in the sugar and then the milk to get a soft dough.
4. Turn on to a floured work surface and knead very lightly. Pat out to a round 2cm/¾in thick. Use a 5cm/2in cutter to stamp out rounds and place on a baking sheet. Lightly knead together the rest of the dough and stamp out more scones to use it all up.
5. Brush the tops of the scones with the beaten egg. Bake for 12-15 minutes until well risen and golden.

4. Quick and Easy pancakes

This really is a quick recipe and can be topped with either sweet or savory foods of your choice.

Serves 2-4
- 1 egg
- 1 cup* of milk
- 1 cup* of flour (any type)
- Cooking oil or butter

* cup = approximately 200ml

Preparation method
1. Place the egg, milk, and flour into a bowl and whisk to combine thoroughly to form a smooth batter.
2. Heat a frying pan until hot then add the sunflower oil or butter and a large spoonful of the pancake mix.
3. Fry over a medium heat until golden brown underneath.
4. Turn the pancake over and cook for a further 1-2 minutes, or

until cooked through and golden brown.
5. Set aside and repeat with the remaining batter.

Serving suggestions

Try with stewed apples or tinned pears, peaches, strawberries or raspberries and serve with single cream (remember tinned fruit is lower in potassium than fresh). For a savory pancake try serving topped with ham, grated cheese or tuna or perhaps a hot filling such as chili (see recipe in the mince section).

Vegetarian Dishes

Worry not if you are a vegetarian, there are various recipes you can enjoy also.

1. **Cauliflower Cheese**

This recipe uses both milk and cheese which may imply that it is high in phosphate and potassium; however, it makes a large amount of cauliflower cheese to serve 4-6 people. Per portion it should contain 25g/1oz of cheese and 125ml/ ¼ pt milk maximum which is within the allowances for those requiring restrictions.

Serves 4-6
- 1 large cauliflower (leaves cut off), broken into pieces
- 500ml milk
- 4 tbsp flour
- 50g (1¾oz) butter
- 100g (3½oz) strong cheddar, grated
- 2-3 tbsp breadcrumbs, if you have them

Preparation method
1. Bring a large saucepan of water to the boil, then add the cauliflower and cook for 5 minutes – lift out a piece to test, it should be cooked. Drain the cauliflower, and then tip into an ovenproof dish.
2. Heat oven to 220°C (200°C Fan)/425°F/Gas 7.
3. Put the saucepan back on the heat and add the milk, flour and butter. Keep whisking fast as the butter melts, and the mixture comes to the boil – the flour will disappear, and the sauce will begin to thicken. Whisk for 2 minutes while the sauce bubbles

and becomes nice and thick. Turn off the heat, stir in most of the cheese and pour over the cauliflower. Scatter over the remaining cheese and breadcrumbs.
4. Bake the Cauliflower cheese in the oven for 20 minutes until bubbling.

Tip: Make enough for 6 portions even if you need less as spare portions can be frozen prior to being baked.

2. Pumpkin Risotto

This is a filling dish and although it contains butternut squash (a vegetable with moderate amounts of potassium), it is made with rice (rather than potatoes) which lowers the potassium content of the overall dish. The cheese used for this recipe is minimal. However, you can enjoy this meal without cheese, making it lower in phosphate and fat.

Serves 3-4
- 570ml (1 pint) vegetable such as low salt Bouillon or chicken stock
- 1 small onion, chopped
- 12 fresh sage leaves, chopped finely
- 2 tbsp olive oil
- 170g (6oz) Arborio (risotto) rice
- 250g (9oz) pumpkin or butternut squash, diced small
- 50g (2oz) butter
- Freshly ground black pepper
- Piece of fresh parmesan, or vegetarian parmesan-style grating cheese (optional)

Preparation method
1. Heat the stock until almost boiling and then simmer over a very low heat. In a separate heavy-based saucepan sweat the onion in the oil until soft but not browned. Add the chopped sage and cook for a couple more minutes.
2. Add the rice and mix well for a few seconds to coat the grains with oil, then pour in one-third of the stock and bring to a gentle simmer. Cook until almost all the stock is absorbed. Add the pumpkin or squash and a little more stock, and continue to

simmer gently until the stock is absorbed.
3. Add the remaining stock a little at a time, until the pumpkin is soft and the rice nicely al dente. You may not need all the stock, but the texture should be loose and creamy.
4. Stir the butter into the risotto, and season well with salt and pepper. Divide into four servings and add grated cheese.

3. Pastry-less Quiche

This is a very versatile recipe in as much as you can easily replace any of the vegetables with any of your favorite vegetable for example peas and dried mint or squash and sage in place of the peppers, mushrooms and tomatoes work well. This dish can also be eaten hot or cold making it great for dinner at home or eaten in a packed lunch. Note that tomatoes and mushrooms are both high potassium foods but ok when eaten in small amounts.

Serves 4
- 1 green pepper, diced
- 1 red pepper, diced
- 1 onion, chopped
- 8 medium mushrooms, sliced
- 2 large or 3 medium tomatoes, sliced
- 5 eggs
- 250g (9oz) fat-free natural cottage cheese
- 75ml milk
- 50g (1¾oz) grated cheddar cheese or use a lower phosphate cheese such as feta

Preparation method
1. Gently fry the prepared vegetables (except the tomatoes) using either a small amount of vegetable oil or a spray oil. You still want them to be a little crunchy, so don't overdo the veg.
2. Mix together the 5 eggs, 250g fat-free natural cottage cheese and the milk – this isn't a pretty mixture but stick with it.
3. Lay the chopped vegetables out in an oven-proof flan dish then pour the cottage cheese mixture over.
4. Placed the sliced tomatoes over the top and sprinkle with the cheese
5. Pop in the oven at 190°C(170°C Fan)/375°F/Gas 5, for around

30-45 minutes, or until the quiche is set and golden brown.

The Versatile Mince Section - for vegetarians too

This whole section has been dedicated to the versatility of mince and includes all kinds of mince; beef pork, lamb, chicken, turkey and vegetarian mince. You can decide which mince you would

prefer to use for each of these recipes. If you are trying to lose weight than opting for the lean or extra lean beef, chicken or turkey mince is best. Alternatively, you may wish to try vegetarian

mince as this is also naturally low fat and a good source of protein.

1. Kidney-Friendly Pasty

These pasties are great served hot from the oven but are equally tasty cold in a packed lunch. It is recommended par-boiling the swede and carrot in this recipe as this helps lower the potassium content of these vegetables.

Makes approximately 6
- 250g (8oz) of your chosen mince
- 1 medium onion, finely chopped
- 1 medium carrot, peeled and chopped
- ½ small swede or ¼ large one, peeled and chopped
- 2 teaspoons dried parsley
- 120ml low salt stock
- ½ teaspoon of English mustard
- 500g (17oz) ready-made shortcrust pastry
- 1 medium egg, lightly whisked
- Pepper

Preparation method
1. Preheat the oven to 180°C (160°C Fan)/350°F/ Gas 4.
2. On the hob boil the chopped swede and carrot for 5-10 minutes or until just slightly soft, then drain and discard the water (this helps lower the potassium content of these vegetables). Allow the vegetable to cool.
3. In a separate bowl add the parsley, stock, onion, minced beef and English Mustard.
4. Use a knife to cut the minced beef into small strands and mix the lot together with your hands so that the ingredients are

roughly spread evenly throughout the mixture. Season with pepper.
5. Add the cooled vegetables and gently combine with your mince mixture.
6. Take the pastry and roll it out with a rolling pin to about 3mm thick. Press a saucer over the rolled pastry and cut around it to leave a circle of pastry. You may need to do three circles then reform and re-roll the pastry. Place some of the fillings on each circle.
7. Brush a small amount of the egg around the edges of the pastry. Bring two edges of the pastry together to make a 'parcel' and crimp the edges together all the way around.
8. Brush the sides of the pasties with the egg (to give a browned color during cooking).
9. Put the pasties in the pre-heated oven on a greased baking tray for 55 minutes.

2. Lasagne

Lasagne generally contains 2 high potassium foods, tomatoes and milk, making it an avoidable dish for those that need to follow a low potassium diet. In this recipe, is used soya milk which creates an equally tasty white sauce but is lower in potassium than cow's milk. You may also wish to top your lasagne with some grated mozzarella cheese, which is a lower phosphate option to cheddar cheese.

Serves 3-4
- 1 tbsp of vegetable or olive oil
- 250g (9oz) of your chosen mince
- 1 onion, diced
- 3 carrots, grated
- 75g (2½oz) butter or low fat spread
- 75g (2½oz) plain flour
- 1 tsp English mustard
- 750ml soya milk
- 2 garlic cloves, crushed
- 1 x 400g (14oz) tin of chopped tomatoes
- 1 low salt stock cube (beef or vegetable)
- 100ml water
- 250g (9oz) lasagne sheets

- 1 tsp oregano or basil (optional)
- Pepper
- 1 large handful of grated mozzarella (optional)

Preparation method
1. Preheat the oven to 200°C (180°C Fan)/400°F/Gas 6
2. Heat a large frying pan over medium heat and add the olive oil or spray oil. Once hot, add the mince of your choice along with a good pinch of pepper. Brown the mince for 5-6 minutes until colored all over and beginning to crisp. Remove the mince from the pan and set to one side.
3. Add the onion and carrot to the frying pan. Cook gently for 10 minutes, or until everything is softened.
4. Meanwhile, melt the butter or spread in a saucepan over a medium heat. Once melted, add the flour and mustard, stir to mix well. Leave to cook over medium heat for two minutes, or until the mixture makes a paste.
5. Pour the soya milk in batches into the saucepan, whisking as you add to create a smooth white sauce. Once all the soya milk is added season with a pinch of black pepper, turn the heat down and leave to simmer very gently for seven minutes.
6. Once the onions and carrots are softened, add the garlic to the frying pan and cook for two minutes. Return the meat (plus any juices) to the pan and add the tomatoes, stock, and water. Mix everything together, cover with a lid and simmer the sauce for 10 minutes until thickened slightly.
7. To assemble the lasagne, place a quarter of the tomato sauce into the bottom of a small/medium baking dish. Top with a layer of lasagna sheets. Spoon over another quarter of the tomato sauce and top with a third of the white sauce. Repeat this twice more, finishing at the top with the last layer of white sauce.
8. If using top, you dish with the grated mozzarella
9. Place into the preheated oven and bake for 30 minutes or until bubbling, and the top is golden brown.

3. Cottage Pie

Those of you on a potassium restriction may be concerned that the topping for this dish contains potato, a high potassium food, however, has been reduced the amount of potato used for this recipe and replaced it with swede, a low potassium food, helping to reduce the overall amount of potassium and make a tasty alternative topping.

Serves 4
- 400g (14oz) potatoes, such as King Edward or Maris Piper, peeled, cut into pieces
- 400g (14oz) swede, peeled, cut into small pieces
- knob of butter or low-fat olive oil spread
- splash of milk
- freshly ground black pepper
- 1 tbsp of vegetable or olive oil
- 1 onion, peeled, finely chopped
- 1 garlic clove, peeled, crushed to a paste with the edge of a knife
- 1 large carrot, peeled, finely chopped
- 1 tin of peas in water
- 2 tsp chopped fresh thyme leaves
- 250-300g (9-11oz) of your chosen mince
- 200ml low salt beef or vegetable stock
- 1 tbsp tomato purée
- Freshly ground black pepper

Preparation method
1. Preheat the oven to 190°C (170°C Fan)/375°F/Gas 5.
2. For the topping, place the potatoes and swede into a large pan of water. Bring to the boil and cook for 15-20 minutes, or until tender. Once cooked, drain ensuring you discard all the water to remove the potassium.
3. Add the butter to the cooked potato and swede and mash using a potato masher or ricer. Add the milk, a little at a time, and continue to mash until smooth. Season, to taste, freshly ground black pepper. Set aside.
4. For the filling, heat the oil in a large pan over a low to medium heat. Add the onion and fry for 8-10 minutes, or until softened.
5. Add the garlic and carrot and fry for a further 4-5 minutes, or until softened.
6. Add your chosen mince to the pan and fry for a further 2-3 minutes, stirring continuously.
7. Add the tomato purée and the stock and stir well to combine.

Bring the mixture to a simmer and continue to simmer for a further 4-5 minutes or until the sauce has thickened. Add the tinned peas and season, to taste, with black pepper
8. Spoon the filling mixture into a large ovenproof dish. Spread the mashed potato and swede mixture over the filling in a smooth, even layer.
9. Transfer to the oven and cook for 18-20 minutes, or until the topping is golden-brown and the filling is cooked through.

4. Spaghetti Bolognese

Spaghetti Bolognese is a classic comfort food and although those on a potassium restriction might avoid it for its tomato and mushroom contents it is, in fact, fine to eat because it is traditionally served with spaghetti, a low potassium food.

Serves 3-4
- 1 tbsp of vegetable or olive oil
- 200g (7oz) of your chosen mince
- 1 onion, finely chopped
- 4 large mushrooms, sliced
- 1 carrot, grated
- 1 400g (14oz) tin of chopped tomatoes
- 230ml of low salt beef or vegetable stock
- 2 tbsp tomato purée
- ½ tsp Worcestershire sauce
- 1 tsp freshly ground black pepper
- 1 tsp of dried basil (optional)
- 300g (10½oz) wholemeal spaghetti

Preparation method
1. Heat the olive oil in a large saucepan over medium heat. Add the mince and the onion and fry for five minutes, stirring occasionally until the mince is browned and the onions softened.
2. Add mushrooms and carrot, cook for around one minute, then add tinned tomatoes, vegetable stock, tomato purée, Worcestershire sauce, freshly ground black pepper, and basil if using. Stir well and bring to the boil, then reduce the heat to simmer for 15-20 minutes, until the sauce has thickened.

3. Place the wholemeal spaghetti in a deep saucepan full of salted boiling water and cook according to packet instructions, then drain.
4. To serve, divide the cooked spaghetti between four dishes, spoon equal portions of Bolognese sauce over each.

5. Chilli Con Carne

This recipe does contain kidney beans which are high in potassium but as this meal is served with rice which is a much lower potassium food than other starchy foods like potatoes then it is fine if you would prefer you can omit the kidney beans and try something different like sweet corn.

Serves 3-4
- 1 tbsp of vegetable or olive oil
- 1 onion, diced
- 2 garlic cloves, chopped
- 250g (9oz) of your chosen mince
- Pepper
- ½ -1 tsp chili flakes, to taste
- 1 x 400g (14oz) tin of chopped tomatoes
- 300ml of low salt beef or vegetable stock
- ½ tsp dried mixed herbs
- ½ tsp of smoked paprika (optional)
- 1 x 400g (14oz) tin red kidney beans, drained and rinsed
- 200g (7oz) long grain rice or basmati rice

Preparation method
1. Heat a large saucepan over medium heat. Add the oil and, once hot, fry the onion for five minutes, or until soft and translucent. Once soft, add the garlic and cook for two minutes.
2. Add the mince, along with a good pinch of pepper. Mix well and cook for 5-6 minutes, or until there are no raw bits of meat. Add the chili flakes, tomatoes, stock, dried mixed herbs and smoked paprika if using. Stir to mix well and bring to a simmer.
3. Pour in the drained kidney beans and simmer gently for 30 minutes, or until the chili con carne is thickened and rich. Taste and adjust the seasoning as necessary.
4. Meanwhile, cook the rice according to the packet instructions.

5. Serve the chili con carne on top of the rice.

Simple Chicken Dishes

All the recipes in this section can be adapted to serve two people rather than four simply by halving the quantities. They also all work well served with potatoes, however for a meal low in potassium serve with rice or pasta. Equally, if you're not a fan of chicken or just fancy a change all these recipes would work well with turkey.

1. Chicken and Leek Pie Filling

This recipe can be used to make a chicken pie with a pastry lid but if you prefer you could use a mash potato topping. For a low potassium topping try swede mashed with a small amount of low salt stock or butter and milk.

Serves 4
- 30g (1oz) unsalted butter
- 30g (1oz) plain flour
- 350ml low salt chicken stock
- 3 tbsp single or double cream
- 500g (1lb 2oz) of leftover roast chicken
- 2 leeks roughly chopped
- 1 packet of ready-made pastry

Preparation method
1. Preheat oven to 180°C (160°C Fan)/350°F/Gas 4.
2. In a saucepan, melt the butter on a low heat and add the flour. Stir until it clumps together and continue cooking and stirring for a couple of minutes. Gradually whisk in the chicken stock a little at a time to avoid lumps. When all the stock is added, allow the sauce to simmer for several minutes and continue stirring until thickened. In another saucepan boil the leeks until tender and drain.
3. Combine the leeks, cream, and chicken with the sauce and decant in to a pie dish. Lightly grease the edges of the dish and top with your chosen pastry recipe. If using pastry crimp or fork around the edges and glaze with a little beaten egg. Bake for 30 minutes or until the topping has colored to a light golden brown.

2. Chicken Wrapped in Pancetta (or Bacon) Stuffed with Herb Cream Cheese

This is a quick and easy recipe that provides a good source of protein. The cream cheese is low in phosphate and if served with rice, pasta or noodles rather than potatoes would also be low in potassium. This recipe would also be tasty served with cranberry sauce (a low potassium sauce).

Serves 4
- 4 large skinless chicken breasts
- 4 tbsp soft cream cheese
- 20 thin slices pancetta or your favorite bacon
- 2 tbsp olive oil
- ½ tsp each of basil/oregano/rosemary/thyme
- Optional cranberry sauce

Preparation method
1. Preheat the oven to 200°C/400°F/Gas 6.
2. In a small bowl, mix the soft cheese with basil, oregano, rosemary and thyme
3. For the chicken, with a small, sharp knife, make an incision down the side of each chicken breast to form a pocket. Season the chicken inside and out with freshly ground black pepper, then push the soft cheese mixture into the pockets. Lightly press each chicken breast to flatten the filling slightly and seal the edges, then wrap each breast in five slices of pancetta, to cover completely.
4. Heat the olive oil in a large, heavy-based frying pan over a medium heat, then add the chicken and fry for 2-3 minutes on each side, or until the pancetta is crisp and golden-brown. Transfer to a roasting tin and cook in the oven for 20-25 minutes, or until the chicken is thoroughly cooked (the juices should be clear with no trace of pink).

3. Chicken and Olive Casserole

This recipe will freeze well so if you're only cooking for 1 or 2 people it is still worth making the full recipe and popping some in the freezer as a homemade ready meal for when you're short on time.

Serves 4
- 1 tbsp of vegetable or olive oil
- 800g (1lb 8oz) chicken breast
- 1 large onion, sliced
- 2 cloves garlic, minced
- 400g tin of chopped tomatoes
- 375ml low salt chicken stock
- 1 tsp dried sage
- ½ tsp dried thyme
- ½ tsp sugar
- 2 tsp balsamic vinegar
- 1 cup olives in brine (black or green or a mixture)
- Pepper

Preparation method
1. Heat a deep pan, spray with oil and brown chicken. Remove chicken from pan and set aside.
2. Add onions and garlic to the pan and sauté until tender. Add tomatoes, chicken stock, sage, thyme, sugar, balsamic vinegar and olives. Bring to the boil and simmer a couple of minutes.
3. Check the seasoning before returning chicken to the pan. Cover and simmer gently for 1 hour.
4. You don't want the casserole to boil as it makes the chicken tough. Just a gentle bubble will give you lovely tender chicken.
5. Serve with boiled rice and vegetables.

4.   Chicken or Vegetarian Curry

This curry is a great low potassium option, and when served with wholemeal rice rather than white rice will be high in fiber. You may want to add some extra vegetables to ensure you get your 5aday, such as green beans (you can even get these frozen). To turn this dish into a vegetarian option simply use a 400g tin of chickpeas to replace the chicken and enjoy. Remember both chicken and chickpeas contain phosphate so if you are prescribed a binder ensure you take as directed with this dish.

Serves 4 Seasoning

Preparation method
1. Combine the seasoning ingredients together in a bowl and then add the chicken or chickpeas to coat.
2. Heat the oil in a large heavy-based saucepan, then add the chicken or chickpeas and cook until sealed.
3. Add the onion and ginger and cook for a further 1-2 minutes.
4. Add the stock, chutney, sugar, and bring to the boil. Cover and simmer for 15 minutes
5. Stir in cream and heat through, taking care not to boil the sauce.
6. Serve with boiled rice, ideally brown rice, and some vegetables.

5. Chicken and Lemon Casserole

This is a lovely recipe that uses the cheaper cuts of chicken making it tasty and economical. If severed with rice and boiled low potassium vegetables such as carrots, cabbage, cauliflower or green beans then the overall potassium content of this dish would below.

Serves 4
- 2 tbsp honey
- 1 lemon, zest, and juice only, plus 1 lemon, sliced into thin rounds
- 2kg (4lb 4oz) skinless chicken thighs or drumsticks
- salt and freshly ground black pepper
- 80g (3oz) butter
- 1 tbsp of vegetable or olive oil
- 4 garlic cloves crushed
- 500ml hot low salt chicken stock
- 2 tsp of dried thyme (optional)

Preparation method
1. Preheat the oven to 200°C (180°C Fan)/400°F/Gas 6.
2. Place the honey, lemon zest, and lemon juice into a bowl and whisk until well combined. Add the chicken pieces and turn until they are completely coated in the mixture. Set aside for at least 10 minutes to marinate.
3. In a flame proof casserole pan heat 40g/1½oz of the butter and half of the olive oil over medium heat. When the butter is foaming, add half of the marinated chicken pieces and fry for 5-6 minutes, turning occasionally, until golden brown. Set the chicken pieces aside and repeat the process with the remaining

butter oil and chicken pieces then set the chicken aside again.
4. Add the garlic cloves, lemon slices, and residual marinade juices to the pan and stir well, scraping any burned bits off the bottom of the pan with a wooden spoon. Return the cooked chicken pieces to the pan, then add the hot chicken stock and the thyme and stir well. Bring the mixture to the boil, place into the oven to cook for 30-35 minutes, or until the chicken is tender and cooked through.
5. Remove the chicken pieces from the pan and set aside on a warm plate. Strain the sauce into a saucepan through a fine sieve, pressing the garlic pulp through the sieve using the back of a wooden spoon. Simmer the lemon sauce over high heat for a further 5-10 minutes, or until the liquid has reduced to the consistency of thin syrup.
6. Spoon the lemon sauce over the casseroled chicken and serve.

Simple Meat Dishes

Lamb and Pork are tasty and versatile meat which can be enjoyed in simple dishes such as these or as part of a stew or even barbequed. Simply served with boiled or mashed potatoes or for a low potassium option couscous or rice and mixed low potassium vegetables such as carrots, broccoli, and peas.

1. Minted Lamb Chops

Although this recipe ideally calls for fresh herbs, you can still make this with any dried herbs you may have lurking in your cupboard; just reduce the quantity by half.

Serves 2
- 100g (3½oz) breadcrumbs (homemade or shop brought)
- 2 tbsp fresh mint
- 1 tbsp fresh parsley
- 2 lamb chops
- 100g (3½oz) flour
- 1 free-range egg, whisked
- 1 tbsp of vegetable or olive oil

Preparation method
1. To prepare the lamb chops, use a blender to mix the

breadcrumbs, mint, and parsley until well combined. Place into a bowl.
2. Coat the lamb chops in the flour then dip in the egg and into the breadcrumbs until well coated. Season with pepper.
3. Heat a frying pan to medium heat. Add the oil and place the lamb chops into the pan. Cook for three minutes.
4. Turn the chops over and cook for a further three minutes.
5. Remove the chops and allow them to rest for three minutes then serve.

2. Honey Glazed Pork or Lamb Chops

Contrasting flavours from the honey and mustard packs a huge amount of taste in this easy to prepare dish. Try marinating the meat overnight to infuse the flavours into the meat.

Serves 2
- 2 lamb or pork chops
- 25g (¾oz) butter or low fat spread
 1 tsp honey
- 1tsp wholegrain mustard
- Black pepper

Preparation method
1. Beat the butter or spread until creamy.
2. Blend in the honey and mustard and season with pepper and mix to a smooth paste
3. Brush the honey mixture over your chosen chop, cover and chill for approximately an hour
4. Grill the chops under a hot grill for 5 minutes each side until cooked and serve

3. Pan-fried Pork Chop with Creamy Leek Sauce

Cream is much lower in potassium and phosphate compared to milk and as such can be enjoyed much more freely on a renal diet (unless you are trying to lose weight, where you might wish to use half fat crème Fraiche instead). Using strong flavours like leek and garlic can help to flavour the foods rather than relying on salt. Serve with a low potassium starchy food like rice or couscous.

Serves 2
- 2 pork chops
- 1 tbsp of vegetable or olive oil
- knob unsalted butter
- 1 garlic clove, peeled and chopped
- ½ leek washed and sliced
- 2 sprigs of thyme, leaves only 50ml milk
- 150ml double cream
- 1 tbsp fresh parsley, chopped with

Preparation method
1. Heat a griddle or frying pan until hot. Brush the pork chop with oil and add to the pan to cook for six minutes. Turn the chop over and cook for a further six minutes, or until browned and cooked through. When cooked, the juices will run clear when pierced with a sharp knife. Remove from the heat and set aside to rest for three minutes.
2. For the leeks, heat the oil and butter in a pan and sauté the garlic
   with the leek and thyme leaves for 3-4 minutes to soften.
3. Stir in the milk, cream, and parsley, then reduce the heat and simmer gently for a further 6-8 minutes, stirring occasionally.
4. Spoon the creamed leek sauce over the pork chop and serve.

4. **Toad in the Hole**

Treating yourself to some good quality sausages from the butchers or deli counter will help to reduce the amount of additives which are frequently added to more processed foods. Adding low potassium flavourings such as mustard is a great way to jazz up the sausages.

Serves 4
- 100g (3½oz) plain flour
- ½ tsp English mustard powder
- 1 egg
- 300ml milk
- 3 thyme sprigs, leaves only (optional)
- 8 sausages
- 2 tbsp of vegetable or olive oil

Preparation method
1. Heat oven to 220°C (200°C Fan)/425°F/Gas 7.
2. Tip the flour into a large mixing bowl and stir in the mustard powder. Make a well in the center, crack in the egg, then pour in a dribble of milk. Stir with a wooden spoon, gradually incorporating some of the flour, until you have a smooth batter in the well. Now add a bit more milk and continue stirring until all the milk and flour has been mixed together.
3. You should now have a smooth, lump-free batter that is the consistency of double cream. Tip it into the jug you measured your milk in, for easier pouring later on, then stir in the thyme if using.
4. Use scissors to snip the links between your sausages, then drop them into a 20 x 30cm roasting tin. Add 1 tbsp of the oil, tossing the sausages in it to thoroughly coat the base of the tin, then roast in the oven for 15 mins.
5. Take the hot tray from the oven, then quickly pour in the batter – it should sizzle and bubble a little when it first hits the hot fat. Put it back into the oven, then bake for 40 mins until the batter is cooked through, well risen and crisp. If you poke the tip of a knife into the batter in the middle of the tray, it should be set, not sticky or runny.

Fish Dishes

Fish is a great source of protein, ideal for replacing any protein lost during dialysis. If cooked with minimal fat, fish is low fat so also ideal if you are trying to lose weight.

1. Fish Pie

You can choose a mixture of all your favorite fish to make this tasty dish and it can be made in advance then heated up in the microwave or made and frozen for another day.

Serves 4
- 300g (11oz) potatoes, peeled and cut into pieces
- 300g (11oz) swede, peeled and cut into pieces
- 1 tbsp of vegetable or olive oil
- 1 onion, finely chopped
- 1 tsp dried mixed herbs (or fresh if available)

- 600g (1lb 3oz) fish pie mix, any bones removed
- 200g (7oz) cream cheese (garlic & herbs flavour)
- Approximately 75ml semi-skimmed milk
- 20g (½oz) cheddar cheese, finely grated

Preparation method
1. Cook the potatoes and swede in boiling water until soft.
2. Meanwhile, heat the oil in a large non-stick frying pan. Add the onion and herbs and cook gently until the onion is soft but not browned.
3. Add the fish to the frying pan and heat until the fish is just cooked through. Add the cream cheese, stir over the heat until the cream cheese has melted and heated up to almost boiling. Gradually add the milk to give a nice creamy sauce. Season with pepper to taste.
4. Spoon the fish mixture into a pre-warmed ovenproof dish. Drain and mash the hot potatoes and swede. Use to top the Fish mixture. Sprinkle with grated cheese and place under a hot grill until the cheese has melted and browned. Serve with seasonal vegetables.

2. Kedgeree

This is a versatile dish which can be served as a main meal, snack or starter.

Serves 4
- 200g (7oz) long-grain rice
- ½ onion finely sliced
- 1 tbsp of vegetable or olive oil
- 2 teaspoons curry powder
- 400g (14oz) poached smoked haddock or cod fillets
- 400ml low salt chicken stock
- 4 hard-boiled eggs
- ½ a lemon

Preparation method
1. Warm the oil in a wide frying pan, add the onion and fry until softened. Add the curry powder and rice and stir to coat the rice in the oil. Add the stock or water, cover with a tight-fitting lid

or tin foil and allow to simmer on a low heat until most of the water has absorbed (around 10 minutes).
2. When most of the water has been absorbed, place the Fish and quartered eggs on top of the rice and replace the lid. Continue to cook on the lowest heat for another few minutes and then turn off the heat leaving the rice, Fish and eggs covered to steam for 5-10 minute with the lid on allowing the Fish to warm through.
3. When the time is up remove the lid and fork the Fish through the rice with a squeeze of lemon juice.

3. Tuna Pasta Bake

This is an ideal recipe for a quick supper, and you may already have all the ingredients in the cupboard/fridge.

Serves 4
- 25g (1oz) unsalted butter or olive oil spread
- ½ tsp mustard or mustard powder
- 25g (1oz) plain flour
- 400ml milk
- 200g (7oz) cream cheese
- Pepper
- ½ onion, peeled, finely chopped
- Handful of each; peas & sweet corn
- 130g (4½oz) canned tuna, drained and flaked
- 160g (5½oz) pasta (such as macaroni, penne or fusilli), cooked according to packet instructions, drained
- 60-80g (2-3oz) dried breadcrumbs (homemade or shop brought)

Preparation method
1. Preheat the oven to 200°C (180°C Fan)/400°F/Gas 6.
2. Heat the butter or spread in a frying pan over a medium heat. When the butter is foaming, add the flour to make a smooth paste. Continue to cook, stirring vigorously, for a further 3-4 minutes, then pour in 125ml/4½fl oz of the milk. Whisk the milk and flour mixture together to a smooth paste.
3. When the mixture is bubbling, add another 125ml/4½fl oz of milk and whisk until it is bubbling and incorporated into the mixture.

4. Repeat the process with the remaining 250ml/9fl oz of milk. Continue to whisk and simmer until the sauce is smooth and thick enough to coat the back of a spoon. Remove the pan from the heat and stir in the cream cheese. Season with pepper and mustard. Add the onion, tuna, peas, sweet corn and cooked pasta to the cheese sauce and stir until well combined.
5. Pour the mixture into an ovenproof dish. Sprinkle over with the breadcrumbs. Bake in the oven for 30 minutes, or until the breadcrumbs are crisp and golden brown, and the sauce is bubbling.

4. Cod fillet with Lemon Sauce

This is a quick and easy dish which can be made with most types of fish including pollock, salmon, plaice, and coley.

Serves 4
- 4 cod fillets
- 1 tbsp cornflour
- 1 tbsp butter or olive oil spread
- 4 tbsp water
- 1 lemon (grated rind and juice)
- Black pepper

Preparation method
1. Place lemon juice and rind into a small saucepan with water and bring to the boil.
2. Mix the cornflour with a little water and add to the saucepan. Cook, stirring continuously until thickened. Add pepper to taste.
3. Dot the Fish with butter (or low fat spread and grill for 5-6 minutes each side until cooked.
4. Serve with our healthy chips or mash, pour over the lemon sauce adding a vegetable of your choice.

5. Easy Fish Cakes

You can make fishcakes from any pre-cooked fish – tinned salmon, tuna or even smoked mackerel. You could also bake a salmon or haddock fillet in the oven from fresh or frozen.

Serves 2-3
- 2 medium potatoes (or sweet potatoes)
- 200g (7oz) cooked flaked Fish, either smoked mackerel or a tin of tuna or salmon
- a small lemon, juice only
- freshly ground black pepper
- 100g (3½oz) cream crackers or similar savory biscuits (or breadcrumbs if you have them)
- 1 tbsp of vegetable or olive oil

Optional extras
- 2 spring onions, chopped
- 1 tbsp chopped chives or parsley
- 1 tbsp grated cheddar
- 1 tsp wholegrain mustard

Preparation method
1. Preheat the oven to 220°C (200°C Fan)/425°F/Gas 7.
2. Peel the potatoes and then boil. After 20-30 minutes the potatoes should feel soft if not, cook them for a few minutes more and then rinse them and leave to cool.
3. Mash the potato using a masher, fork, or clean fingers.
4. Add the fish and mix well. Add the lemon, a little pepper and any of the optional extras you like. Have a taste – you can add more pepper or lemon, if you like.
5. Place the crackers in a sandwich bag and wrap it in a clean tea towel or layers of kitchen paper. Crush the crackers using a rolling pin. Pour the cracker crumbs onto a plate.
6. Get your hands a little bit wet and roll small balls of the Fishcake mixture. Don't worry too much about making perfect balls – you can flatten them into patties. Get the outside of the Fishcakes damp again and push them into the bowl of crushed crackers – you want a light coating of crumbs all over the Fishcakes.
7. Pour the oil over the bottom of a baking tray and place the Fishcakes on top. Turn them all over once so that they have a little oil on each side.
8. Bake the Fishcakes for 10 minutes on one side and then turn the Fishcakes over before placing them back in the oven for

another 10 minutes or until the Fishcakes are golden brown. Carefully remove from the oven and leave to cool slightly before serving.

Side Dishes

1. Healthy Chips

Because these chips are parboiled, they are lower in potassium so great if you're a low potassium diet – plus they are healthy if you use less oil, so the spray oil is great if you are trying to lose weight.

Serves 4
- 908g (2lb) medium sized Maris Piper potatoes
- A small amount of vegetable, olive oil or spray oil

Preparation method
1. Preheat the oven to 240°C (220°C Fan)/475°F/Gas 9. Peel the potatoes using a potato peeler and remove any blemishes or "eyes". Slice lengthwise into approx ½in/1cm thick rectangular chips.
2. Bring a large saucepan of salted water to the boil. Add the chips and cook for 4 minutes. Drain and leave aside for 10 minutes to dry.
3. Return the chips to the dry saucepan, cover with a lid and shake to "rough up" the edges of the chips - this roughness is important to the texture of the chips.
4. Light grease a metal baking tray with olive oil or spray oil. Transfer the chips to the tray, cover lightly with olive oil or spray lightly with oil spray and bake in the oven for 20-25 minutes, turning occasionally, until golden brown on all sides. Drain them on absorbent kitchen paper and serve.

2. Dauphinoise Potatoes

These creamy, garlicky potatoes make a fabulous side dish for any of the meat or poultry dishes. They are very high calorie so best avoided if you are trying to lose weight. Parboiling these potatoes helps to reduce the amount of potassium in this dish.

Serves 4-6
- 1kg (2lb 4oz) potatoes peeled and chopped
- 3-4 cloves garlic
- 500ml (17½fl oz) double cream (you may need a bit extra)
- Freshly ground black pepper
- ½ teaspoon of freshly grated nutmeg (optional)
- 85-100g (4oz) grated cheddar cheese (optional)

Preparation method
1. Preheat the oven to 180°C/350°F/Gas 4.
2. On the hob boil the potatoes for approximately 10 minutes or until slightly soft but still firm on the inside.
3. Drain and discard the cooking water and allow the potatoes to cool.
4. Once cooled, slice the potatoes into thin slices. Place the slices into a bowl as you cut them.
5. Finely slice the garlic or use a garlic press and add to the potatoes.
6. Season the potatoes with ground black pepper and the grated nutmeg if using.
7. Pour the cream over the potatoes and mix well but be gentle so not to turn the potatoes into a mash.
8. Place the potato slices into the gratin dish. They should come to just below the top of the dish. Press the potato down with the back of a spoon or your hands, so it forms a solid layer. The cream should come to just below the top layer of potato (top up with more double cream if necessary).
9. Sprinkle over the grated cheese if using.
10. Place the potatoes in the oven and bake for 30-40 minutes, or until golden brown on the top.

3. Healthy Creamed/Mash Potato

This healthy mashed potato uses clever substitutions to reduce fat and calories but maintain a rich creaminess.

Serves 4
- 1kg (2lbs) floury potatoes, such as King Edward or Maris Piper, cut into even chunks
- 125ml skimmed, 1% or semi-skimmed milk

- 1 tbsp low fat spread
- 3 tbsp low fat crème fraiche

Preparation method
1. Bring a large saucepan of water to the boil. Add the potatoes and boil for about 15 minutes or until tender. Transfer to a colander and drain well, then return to the pan and set over a very low heat for 2 minutes to dry completely.
2. Heat the milk and butter in a small pan, then pour over the potatoes. Remove pan from the heat, then mash potatoes using an electric hand whisk or potato masher. Tip in the crème fraîche and beat with a wooden spoon until smooth and creamy. Season with pepper and a pinch of salt.

4. High Energy Creamy Mash Potato

This is a great alternative to our healthy mash as it provides extra energy without the quantity for those that need to gain weight and build-up.

Serves 4
- 1kg (2lbs) potatoes, cut into large chunks
- 100 ml single cream
- 50g (2oz) unsalted butter, diced
- 50ml double cream
- Freshly grated nutmeg, to taste

Preparation method
1. Boil the potatoes in a large pan of boiling water for 15-20 minutes or until tender. Drain the potatoes in a colander.
2. Meanwhile, pour the single cream into a pan and add the butter, double cream, nutmeg.
3. Pass the cooked potatoes through a potato ricer or mash into a clean bowl.
4. Gradually mix the milk mixture into the potatoes – you may not need it all as you don't want to make the mixture too wet. Beat with a wooden spoon until fluffy and smooth, and then reheat if necessary.

Puddings and Cakes

We all enjoy a sweet treat occasionally. Remember to limit your portion sizes of these if you are trying to losing weight. Many of these recipes have a high sugar content if you have diabetes you may wish to try cutting the amount of sugar or using a granulated sweetener. For people with diabetes small amounts of high sugar foods are best taken with a meal to slow down the absorption of sugar. It is nice to have something to accompany desserts but custard whether homemade or made using custard powder is very high in phosphate, therefore if you are on a phosphate restriction try these alternatives:

- Cream, clotted, single or double are fine but beware if you are trying to lose weight.
- Créme fraîche or low fat/fat-free fromage frais are lighter alternatives to cream.
- Soya ice cream is lower in phosphate than the dairy alternative.

1. Syrup Sponge Pudding

This recipe is good for giving you extra calories but has a high sugar content so take care if you have diabetes. It is however low in both potassium, and phosphate. For a change replace the syrup with Jam.

Serves 4
- 100g (3½oz) softened unsalted butter
- 100g (3½oz) caster sugar
- 2 eggs
- 100g (3½oz) self-raising flour
- 6 tbsp golden syrup

Preparation method
1. Cream the butter and sugar together in a bowl or food processor.
2. Add one egg and mix carefully with a spoon of flour to prevent curdling. Add the other egg and mix well.
3. Fold in the flour.
4. Measure the syrup into a buttered pudding dish. Spoon the cake mixture on top of the syrup.
5. Cover with buttered foil with a fold to allow for expansion.
6. Bake at 200°C (180°C Fan)/400°F/Gas 6 for 35-40 minutes until a skewer comes out clean.

2. Rice Pudding

This recipe uses Soya milk in place of cow's milk as this is lower in phosphate but tastes just as good. If you need to gain weight then you could add some jam, honey or syrup to the finished dish for extra calories.

Serves 6
- 200g (7oz) pudding rice
- 800ml soya milk (used unsweetened one)
- 4 tablespoons sugar
- ½ teaspoon salt
- ½ teaspoon vanilla extract, or to taste
- ¼ teaspoon cinnamon powder (optional)
- ¼ teaspoon nutmeg powder (optional)

Preparation method
1. Add the soya milk and rice to a large pan and stir whilst you bring to the boil.
2. Once boiled reduce the heat and simmer for 20 minutes or until the rice is very soft.
3. Add the sugar, vanilla extract, and salt and cook for another 2 minutes, stirring occasionally.
4. Pour the rice pudding into serving dishes and sprinkle with nutmeg or cinnamon if using.
5. Serve the rice pudding immediately (hot) or cool down and serve cold.

3. Apple Crumble

Apples are not high in potassium and can be added to your crumble or pie without problems. For a low phosphate, option serve with cream rather than custard or a low-fat créme fraîche.

Serves 4
For the crumble
- 300g (10½oz) plain flour, sieved pinch
of salt
- 175g (6oz) sugar
- 200g (7oz) unsalted butter, cubed at

room temperature
- Knob of butter for greasing

For the filling
- 450g (1lb) apples, peeled, cored and cut into 1cm/½in pieces
- 50g (2oz) sugar
- 1 tbsp plain flour
- 1 pinch of ground cinnamon

Preparation method:
1. Preheat the oven to 180°C (160°C Fan)/350°F/Gas 4.
2. Place the flour and sugar in a large bowl and mix well. Taking a few cubes of butter at a time rub into the flour mixture. Keep rubbing until the mixture resembles breadcrumbs.
3. Place the fruit in a large bowl and sprinkle over the sugar, flour and cinnamon. Stir well, being careful not to break up the fruit.
4. Butter a 24cm/9in ovenproof dish. Spoon the fruit mixture into the bottom, then sprinkle the crumble mixture on top.
5. Bake in the oven for 40-45 minutes until the crumble is browned and the fruit mixture bubbling.

4. Lemon Cheesecake

The following recipe is easy to adapt into a fruit cheesecake just by reducing the amount of lemon and then adding any drained tinned fruit on the top. Soft cheeses, such as cream cheese, tend to be lower in phosphate making them suitable for people on a phosphate restriction.

Serves 6
For the base
- 200g (7oz) digestive biscuits
- 100g (3½oz) soft unsalted butter

For the topping
- 1 packet cream cheese (a standard packet normally around 200-300g)
- 1 tub single cream (or whipping cream, a small tub)
- 250g (9oz) icing sugar (sifted)
- Juice of 1 lemon

Preparation method:
1. Whizz the biscuits in the food processor until you have fine crumbs, then add the butter in smallish chunks through the nozzle while the processor is still running. You should end up with a damp dough-like consistency.
2. Butter a tin and press the base mixture down hard into the bottom of the tin, put in the fridge to set.
3. Beat the cream until it is thickened enough to nearly hold it's shape but not quite. Use an electric whisk if you have one to save time.
4. Beat in the packet of cream cheese until the mixture is smooth.
5. Add the sifted icing sugar and lemon juice and beat again until you achieve a smooth thick consistency.
6. Pour topping onto the base and spread, put the tin back into the fridge until the topping has set. Add fruit as preferred.

5. Cherry Shortbread

Shortbread is a low potassium and low phosphate treat as well as being relatively easy to make.

Makes approximately 20 shortbread fingers
- 125g (4oz) unsalted butter
- 55g (2oz) caster sugar, plus extra to fnish
- 180g (6oz) plain flour
- Optional: 2 tbsp glace cherries – chopped

Preparation method
1. Heat the oven to 190°C (170°C Fan)/375°F/Gas 5.
3. Beat the butter and the sugar together until smooth.
4. Stir in the flour to get a smooth paste.
5. Add the cherries (if using) and stir gently to combine.
6. Turn on to a work surface and gently roll out until the paste is 1cm/½in thick.
7. Cut into rounds or fingers and place onto a baking tray. Sprinkle with caster sugar and chill in the fridge for 20 minutes.
8. Bake in the oven for 15-20 minutes, or until pale golden-brown. Set aside to cool on a wire rack.

6. Victoria Sponge Cake

Cakes without nuts, dried fruit, chocolate, and coconut are good choices as they are generally low in potassium and phosphate. Enjoy as a treat!

Serves 10
- 250g (9oz) unsalted butter, well softened
- 250g (9oz) caster sugar
- 4 medium eggs
- 250g (9oz) self-raising flour
- A splash of milk (if required)
- 50ml double cream
- Approximately 5 tbsp raspberry jam (add more or less for your preferred taste)

Preparation method
1. Grease two 20cm shallow cake tins and then line with baking parchment. Preheat the oven to 180°C (160°C Fan)/350°F/Gas 4.
2. Put the softened butter and sugar in a large bowl and beat until very pale and fluffy. This is likely to take between 5-10 minutes. If preferred this can be done in a free-standing mixer.
3. Add an egg and a large spoon of flour to the mixture and beat again. Repeat this process until all the eggs are incorporated. Sift in the remaining flour and fold into the mixture using a large metal spoon.
4. If the mixture does not have a dropping consistency (i.e., drops easily off a spoon) add a splash of milk.
5. Divide the mixture between the two tins, smooth the top and bake in the oven for 25 minutes.
6. When the cakes have cooked and cooled, they can be sandwiched together. Whisk the double cream until soft peaks form. Spread jam on the top of one of the cakes and then spread the whipped cream on top of the jam. Set the second cake on top and sift over icing sugar to decorate.

7. Quick and Easy Flapjacks

The oats in flapjacks are high in soluble fiber but watch out for all the added sugar. For a change, try adding glacé cherries or dried cranberries.

Makes 12
- 250g (9oz) porridge oats
- 125g (4oz) melted unsalted butter
- 125g (4oz) brown sugar
- 2-3 tbsps golden syrup (depends how gooey you want it)

Preparation method
1. Place all the ingredients in a food processor or large bowl and fully   mix, making sure the oats keep their texture.
2. Lightly grease a baking tin with butter and spoon in all the mixture.
3. Using the back of a spoon press into the corners, so the mixture is flat and score the mixture into 12 squares.
4. Place in the oven and bake on 180°C (160°C Fan)/350°F/Gas 4, until golden brown (about 20 minutes).

8. Madeira Cake
Plain cakes are low in both potassium and phosphate so enjoy for an   afternoon tea!

Serves 6-8
- 175g (6oz) unsalted butter, at room temperature
- 175g (6oz) caster sugar
- 3 eggs
- 250g (9oz) self-raising flour
- 2-3 tbsp milk
- 1 lemon, zest only

Preparation method
1. Preheat the oven to 180°C (160°C Fan)/350°F/Gas 4.
2. Grease an 18cm/7in round cake tin, line the base with greaseproof   paper and grease the paper.
3. Cream the butter and sugar together in a bowl until pale and fluffy.
4. Beat in the eggs, one at a time, beating the mixture well between each one and adding a tablespoon of the flour with the last egg to   prevent the mixture curdling.

5. Sift the flour and gently fold in, with enough milk to give a mixture that falls slowly from the spoon. Fold in the lemon zest.
6. 6. Spoon the mixture into the prepared tin and lightly level the top. Bake on the middle shelf of the oven for 30-40 minutes, or until golden brown on top and a skewer inserted into the center comes out clean.

Christmas Recipes

We all would love to try out a new recipe during festive seasons, as neighbors and family would come visiting below are some great recipes.

1.Brie and Cranberry Filo Parcels

Whether you need a tasty starter for your Christmas dinner or some bites to keep party guests going, these cheesy festive morsels will go down a treat! The brie and camembert cheeses are much lower in phosphate than pate or prawns, so if you need to restrict your phosphate, these really help.

Makes: 12 parcels
- 200g pack filo pastry
- 200g brie or camembert cut into 12 even pieces
- 100g cranberry sauce
- 50g salted butter, melted
- Baking sheet lined with baking parchment

Preparation Method
1. Preheat oven to 190C
2. Cut filo pastry into 36 squares measuring 8cm x 8cm. Keep covered with a damp tea towel.
3. For each parcel, take 3 squares of filo, brush each piece with melted butter and arrange on top of each other at an angle to form a star. Place 1 piece of the cheese and a teaspoon of cranberry sauce in the center of the star. Draw the edges of the filo up to form a parcel. Brush with melted butter.
4. Place on prepared baking sheet in preheated oven for 6 to 10 minutes, until crisp and golden.

2. Pitta Crisps with Tzatziki Dip

Pitta bread is a tasty alternative to potato crisps as it is low in potassium

Ingredients
- 4 pitta breads
- 2 tablespoons of olive oil

For dip
- 1 small pot of low-fat plain yogurt
- 1 teaspoon of mint sauce
- 70g of cucumber finely diced

Preparation Method
1. Preheat the oven to 170C (gas 3)
2. Brush each pitta bread on both sides with olive oil. Tear or cut each pitta bread into 6-8 pieces and spread out on a baking tray.
3. Bake the pitta bread for about 20 minutes or until crisp and lightly browned. Leave them to cool on a wire rack
4. Mix the yogurt, mint sauce, and cucumber in a bowl to make the dip.

2. Salmon and Chive Paté
Ingredients
- 200g tin salmon, drained/boned
- 100g soft white cheese spread, e.g., Philadelphia
- 2 tablespoons chopped chives
- 1/4pt (150ml) mayonnaise
- 2 tablespoons lemon juice
- 50g melted margarine

Preparation Method
1. Blend the salmon, soft cream cheese, mayonnaise, and lemon juice until combined. Gradually add the melted margarine and blend till smooth.
2. Stir in the chives. Pour into ramekins and refrigerate.

In brief

Fluid, salt and potassium are the most important considerations. Take special care if you are on a fluid restriction. All drinks (hot, cold and alcoholic), soups, fruit juices, jellies, ice cream and ice lollies must be included in your total daily allowance.

An average portion of soup = 250ml
An average jelly = 150ml
An average ice cream scoop = 75ml
An average ice cube = 25ml

Try to avoid salty snacks, e.g., nuts, crisps, etc. These will make you more thirsty. Take special care if you are on a potassium restriction. Many seasonal foods and drinks are high in potassium, and it would be easy to reach a hazardous intake if care was not taken, particularly at social events. Make sure you read this booklet carefully and telephone us if you have any worries.

4. Sausage & Cranberry Stuffing

Chestnut Stuffing is high in both potassium and phosphate so instead, try these yummy Cranberry & Sausage Stuffing Balls

Ingredients
- 1 onion, finely chopped
- 25g butter
- 2 slices wholemeal bread, whizzed to chunky breadcrumbs
- 200g of lean sausage meat
- 1 apple, peeled & grated
- 200g cranberries, roughly chopped
- 4 sage leaves, finely sliced
- ½ tsp mixed spice

Preparation Method
1. 1. Preheat the oven to 200C, 180C fan, gas 6. Cook the onion in the butter until soft but not browned. Add the breadcrumbs and stir so they soak up all the excess butter. Let the mixture cool. Tip into a bowl with the sausage meat, apple, cranberries, sage, and mixed spice. Mix well, and then roll into balls. You can now cover and chill for up to a day before cooking.
2. To cook, place in a roasting tin and bake for 40 minutes,

turning a few times, or until browned all over.
3. Serve and enjoy as part of your Christmas dinner.

5. Turkey and Apple Curry

Curries are a great way to use up leftover meats from the Christmas meals but some curries can be high in potassium – try this delicious kidney friendly Turkey & Apple Curry

Ingredients
- 500g Turkey leftovers
- 1/2 tsp black pepper
- 2 medium apples, peeled and chopped
- 1 garlic glove, minced
- 3 tbsp butter
- 1 tbsp curry powder
- ½ tbsp. Dried basil
- 3 tbsp all-purpose flour
- 1 cup low sodium chicken stock
- 1 cup rice milk, unsweetened
- Handful fresh coriander

You will need: preheated oven – 180 degrees

Preparation Method
1. In a saucepan or casserole dish, sauté apple, onion, garlic in the butter over a medium heat
2. Add curry powder and basil, mix well and sauté for a further minute
3. Stir in the flour, continue to cook for one minute
4. Add chicken stock, and rice milk, stirring well. Remove from heat.
5. Add turkey leftovers and coriander and heat until piping hot.
6. Serve with boiled green beans and boiled pilau, basmati or plain rice.

6. Jammy Sponge Tarts

Mince Pies are very high in potassium so try these yummy alternatives.

Ingredients
- 200g (7oz) sweet dessert pastry

- (home-made or shop-bought)
- For the topping
- 100g (4oz) butter, softened
- 100g (4oz) caster sugar
- 2 medium eggs
- 75g (3oz) self-raising flour, sifted
- 25g (1oz) semolina
- 4tbsp strawberry jam
- Icing sugar, or dusting

You will need: A greased bun tin, large enough to hold 12 tarts

Preparation Method
1. Preheat the oven to 190C, 170C fan, gas 5. Roll out the pastry on a lightly floured surface and cut into 12x7.5cm (43/4 x3in) fluted rounds, re-rolling the trimmings as required. Use to line the bun tin, then place in the fridge to chill.
2. To prepare the topping, beat together the butter and caster sugar until pale and light. Gradually beat in the eggs, then fold in the flour and semolina. Add a little jam to the pastry cases, then add the topping. Bake for 15 to 20 minutes or until puffed up, golden and set. Leave the tarts to cool in the tin for 5 minutes. Dust with the icing sugar before serving.
3. You can serve with cream such as single, double, or clotted.

7. Christmas Cake

This recipe uses tinned peaches, tinned pineapple, cherries and mixed peel as a low potassium alternative to dried fruit.

Ingredients
- 200g Glace cherries halved
- 200g mixed peel
- 100g tinned peaches, drained and roughly chopped
- 100g tinned pineapple drained and roughly chopped
- 2 eggs, beaten
- 1 tbsp brandy
- 250g plain flour
- 150g self-raising flour
- 200g unsalted butter

- 150g caster sugar
- 1 tsp nutmeg
- 2 tsp mixed spice

Preparation Method
1. Preheat the oven to 150°C/300°F/Gas 4.
2. Grease and line a 7in baking tin.
3. Cream butter and sugar until light and fluffy. Sieve the flour and spices together. Add the eggs and flour alternately to the creamed mixture, mixing well after each addition. Stir in the fruit, peel and brandy. Turn into the tin and cook for 3hours.
4. Ice when cool with white icing but avoid marzipan which is high in
    phosphate.

8. Gingerbread Buche de Noel

Christmas cake and Christmas pudding at both very high in potassium so   why not try making this delicious low potassium ginger log.

Ingredients
- 50g butter, plus extra for greasing
- 50g treacle
- 50g golden syrup
- 2 balls stem ginger finely grated,
- plus 2 tbsp of the syrup
- 4 large eggs
- 100g dark muscovado sugar, plus extra for dusting
- 100g plain flour
- ½ tsp baking powder
- 2 tsp ground ginger
- ½ tsp ground cinnamon
- For the icing
- 200g butter softened
- 250g icing sugar
- 2 tsp vanilla extract
- 3 tbsp ginger syrup from the stem ginger jar

Preparation Method
1. Heat oven to 190C/170C fan/gas 5. Grease and line a 20 x 30cm Swiss roll tin with baking parchment, then grease the parchment a little too. Put the treacle, syrup, butter and stem ginger in a pan, heat until melted and stir to combine, then set aside to cool a little.
2. Put the eggs and sugar in a bowl and whisk using an electric hand whisk until light, mousse-like and doubled in size – this will take about 10 minutes. Sift over the flour, baking powder, and spices, and then pour the melted butter mixture around the sides of the bowl so that it trickles down into the whisked eggs. Very gently fold everything together with a large metal spoon. When just combined pour the mixture into the Swiss roll tin and ease it into the corners. Bake for 12 minutes until just cooked.
3. While the sponge is cooking, place a sheet of baking parchment that is big enough to fit the cake on your work plain and dust with just a little bit of sugar. Once cooked, gently tip the cake directly onto the parchment. Use a small serrated knife to score a line just about 2cm from one of the shorter ends, making sure you don't cut all the way through to the end – this will help to get a tight roll. Gently roll up from this end, rolling the parchment between the layers. Leave to cool to a low temperature like this on a wire rack to help set the shape.
4. To make the icing, put the ingredients in a bowl and whisk until smooth. Transfer to a piping bag that is well fitted with a big round nozzle or use a plastic sandwich bag and cut off one corner to make a hole that is about 1cm wide. Unroll the sponge and drizzle the surface with 2 tbsp ginger syrup. Pipe a layer of ginger buttercream over the inside of the roll, then use the paper underneath to aid in tightly re-rolling it into a roulade. Slice off both ends for a clean finish. The Buche can be frozen. Defrost at room temperature before continuing.
5. Place the Buche on a serving plate or board. Use the remaining icing to pipe a thick layer over the top of the sponge, zigzagging backward and forwards to create a tight concertina pattern. Decorate with white pearl sprinkles, if you like. The Buche will keep in a sealed container for up to 5 days, or can be frozen for up to two months.

9. Christmas Pudding

Ingredients
- 100g self-raising flour
- 100g tinned pineapple chunks (drained and rinsed)
- 100g mixed peel
- 100g glace cherries
- 75g dried cranberries
- 75g tinned plums (drained and chopped)
- 50g porridge oats
- 50g vegetable suet
- 50g dark brown sugar
- 1 tbsp brandy
- 2 eggs, beaten
- 2 teaspoons mixed spice

Preparation Method
1. Grease a 1 liter (2 pint) pudding dish.
2. Mix together the fruit, porridge oats, and suet, stir in the brandy.
3. Add the flour, sugar, and spice, stir in the eggs.
4. Pour the mixture in the pudding bowl and cover with greaseproof paper, secured with string.
5. Cover the greaseproof with foil, again securing the string.
6. Steam for 4 hours over a pan of hot water or using a steamer.
7. Cool and keep in the fridge for up to one week. Steam for a further hour or microwave for 10 minutes before serving.
8. Serve with brandy butter or double cream.

Main renal diet dishes (full dish) with nutritional benefits

It must be known that following a renal diet is not a bad thing. Below we would see lot of main dishes that can be enjoyed while keeping your kidney healthy.

Chili Rice With Beef
Ingredients
2 tablespoons vegetable oil
1 pound lean ground beef
1 cup onion, chopped

2 cups rice, cooked
1 ½ teaspoons chili con carne seasoning powder
⅛ teaspoon black pepper
½ teaspoon sage

Preparation Method
1. Heat oil; add beef and onion. Cook, stirring occasionally until browned.
2. Add rice and seasonings. Mix together.
3. Remove from heat. Cover and let stand 10-14 minutes.

Nutritional content per serving
360 calories 1 grams trans fat 78 milligrams sodium 23 grams protein 65 milligrams cholesterol 427 milligrams potassium 14 grams total fat 26 grams carbohydrate 233 milligrams phosphorus 4 grams saturated fat 2 grams fiber 34 milligrams calcium

Suggestions
- May substitute ground beef with ground turkey or chicken.
- May add ¼ cup chopped green pepper and/or celery.
- May add any of the following seasonings: thyme, garlic powder, onion powder, white pepper, red pepper, oregano, or lemon pepper.
- May substitute 2 cups cooked pasta for rice. Toss pasta in browned beef and seasonings. Remove from heat and serve.

Yield: 4 servings
Serving size: 1 cup

Salisbury Steak
Ingredients
1 pound chopped steak or lean ground beef, chicken or turkey
1 small onion, chopped
½ cup green pepper, chopped
1 teaspoon black pepper
1 egg
1 tablespoon vegetable oil
½ cup water
1 tablespoon corn starch

Preparation Method
1. Mix together meat, onion, green pepper, black pepper, and egg. Form into patties.
2. Heat oil in skillet, add patties and cook on both sides.
3. Add half of water and simmer for 15 minutes. Remove patties.
4. To meat drippings, add remaining water and corn starch. Simmer while stirring
   to thicken gravy.
5. Pour gravy over steak and serve hot.

Nutritional content per serving
249 calories 0 grams trans fat 128 milligrams sodium 22 grams protein 149 milligrams cholesterol 366 milligrams potassium 57 grams total fat 7 grams carbohydrate 218 milligrams phosphorus 3 grams saturated fat 1 gram fibers 33 milligrams calcium
Yield: 4 servings
Serving size: 3-ounces

Parsley Burger
Ingredients
1 pound lean ground beef or ground turkey
1 tablespoon lemon juice
1 tablespoon parsley flakes
¼ teaspoon black pepper
¼ teaspoon ground thyme
¼ teaspoon oregano

Preparation Method
1. Mix all ingredients thoroughly.
2. Shape into 4 small patties about ¾" thick.
3. Place on lightly greased skillet or broiler pan.
4. Broil about 3" from the heat for 10-15 minutes, turning once.

Nutritional content per serving
171 calories 0 grams trans fat 108 milligrams sodium 20 grams protein 90 milligrams cholesterol 289 milligrams potassium 10 grams total fat 0 grams carbohydrate 180 milligrams phosphorus 3 grams saturated fat 0 grams fiber 21 milligrams calcium

Yield: 4 servings
Serving size: 1 patty, 3-ounces

Swedish Meatballs
Ingredients for sauce
¼ cup vegetable oil
2 tablespoons all-purpose flour
1 teaspoon onion powder
2 teaspoons vinegar
2 teaspoons sugar
1 teaspoon Tabasco® sauce
2-3 cups water

Directions for sauce
1. Combine oil and flour in saucepan; stir while cooking until golden brown. Remove from heat.
2. Add onion powder, vinegar, sugar, Tabasco® sauce, and water.
3. Return to heat, and continue stirring until thickened.

Nutritional content per serving
76 calories 0 grams trans fat 31 milligrams sodium 5 grams protein 21 milligrams cholesterol 70 milligram potassium 6 grams total fat 2 grams carbohydrate 44 milligrams phosphorus 1 grams saturated fat 0 grams fiber 7 milligrams calcium
Yield: 35 meatballs
Serving size: 2 meatballs

Ingredients for meatballs
1 pound lean ground beef or turkey
¼ cup onions, finely chopped
1 tablespoon lemon juice
1 teaspoon poultry seasoning (without salt)
1 teaspoon black pepper
¼ teaspoon dry mustard
¾ teaspoon onion powder
1 teaspoon Italian seasoning
1 teaspoon granulated sugar
1 teaspoon Tabasco® sauce

Directions for meatballs
1. Preheat oven to 425°F.
2. Mix all ingredients together well.
3. Shape meatballs by using one tablespoon meat mixture for each meatball.
4. Place meatballs in a baking dish and bake for 20 minutes or until well done. Make the sauce (recipe below).
5. Remove meatballs from oven and combin with sauce. Keep warm until ready to serve.

Open-Faced Steak & Onion Sandwich
Ingredients
4 chopped steaks (4-ounces each)
1 tablespoon lemon juice
1 tablespoon Italian seasoning
1 tablespoon black pepper
1 tablespoon vegetable oil
1 medium onion, sliced into rings
4 hoagie rolls, sliced

Preparation Method
1. Combine meat with lemon juice, Italian seasoning, and black pepper.
2. Heat oil in frying pan over medium heat.
3. Brown seasoned steaks on both sides until tender. Remove and drain on paper towels.
4. Lower heat; add onion and sauté until onions are tender.
5. Serve open-faced on sliced hoagie roll, topped with onion rings.

Nutritional content per serving
345 calories 0 grams trans fat 247 milligrams sodium 14 grams protein 40 milligrams cholesterol 200 milligrams potassium 21 grams total fat 26 grams carbohydrate 115 milligrams phosphorus 7 grams saturated fat 2 grams fiber 98 milligrams calcium

Suggestions
• May be prepared in oven using cooking spray for oil. Bake for 30-

45 minutes at 400°F.
- May be served on herb bread*.
- May use lean ground beef, turkey or chicken as a substitute.
- May use other seasonings: thyme, basil, bay leaf, caraway seeds, savory, oregano, green pepper, garlic powder, onion powder, liquid smoke.

*Recipe included – see index
Yield: 4 servings
Serving size: 3-ounces

Taco Stuffing
Ingredients
2 tablespoon vegetable oil
1 ¼ pounds lean ground beef or turkey
½ teaspoon ground red pepper
½ teaspoon black pepper
1 teaspoon Italian seasoning
1 teaspoon garlic powder
1 teaspoons onion powder
½ teaspoon Tabasco® sauce
½ teaspoon nutmeg
Will also need:
1 medium taco shells
½ head shredded lettuce

Preparation Method
1. 1. Heat oil. Place ground meat and all remaining ingredients except taco shells and lettuce in a skillet. Cook until beef is done and ingredients are well-blended.
2. Stuff taco shells with 2-ounces of meat and top with shredded lettuce.

Nutritional content per serving
(Includes taco shell and shredded lettuce)
176 calories 0 grams trans fat 124 milligrams sodium 14 grams protein 56 milligrams cholesterol 258 milligrams potassium 9 grams total fat 9 grams carbohydrate 150 milligrams phosphorus 2 grams saturated fat 0 grams fiber 33 milligrams calcium
Yield: 8 servings

Serving size: 2-ounces stuffing in each shell

Basic Meat Loaf
Ingredients
1 pound lean ground turkey
1 egg white
1 tablespoon lemon juice
½ cup plain bread crumbs
½ teaspoon onion powder
½ teaspoon Italian seasoning
¼ teaspoon black pepper
½ cup chopped onions
½ cup diced green bell pepper
¼ cup water

Preparation Method
1. Preheat oven to 400°F.
2. Pour lemon juice over meat.
3. In a bowl, combine remaining ingredients.
4. Add to meat and mix well.
5. Place in a loaf pan; bake for 45 minutes.

Nutritional content per serving
110 calories 0 grams trans fat 71 milligrams sodium 12 grams protein 42 milligrams cholesterol 138 milligrams potassium 5 grams total fat 2 grams carbohydrate 87 milligrams phosphorus
1 grams saturated fat 0 grams fiber 20-milligram calcium

Suggestions
• May add carrot and celery.
• May substitute bread crumbs with crushed crackers, toasted white bread crumbs   or cornflakes.
Yield: 8 servings
Serving size: 2-ounces

Turkey & Noodles
Ingredients
2 cups dry elbow macaroni
1 tablespoon vegetable or olive oil

2 pounds fresh lean ground turkey
½ cup green onions, chopped
½ cup green pepper, chopped
1 14-ounce can regular diced tomatoes
1 tablespoon Italian seasoning
1 teaspoon black pepper

Preparation Method
1. 1. Cook macaroni in medium boiler in 4 cups of boiling water. Allow to boil for 5 minutes or desired tenderness. Drain and set a side.
2. Heat vegetable oil in a large skillet over medium heat. Add ground turkey and cook until done, stirring occasionally.
3. Add onions, green peppers, diced tomatoes, Italian seasoning, black pepper and cooked macaroni. Mix well.
4. Cover and let simmer for 5 minutes or until desired. Serve warm.

Nutritional content per serving
273 calories 0 grams trans fat 188 milligrams sodium 33 grams protein 80 milligrams cholesterol 533 milligrams potassium 7 grams total fat 22 grams carbohydrates 296 milligrams phosphorus 1 grams saturated fat 2 grams fibers 55 milligrams calcium

Suggestions
• May use other vegetables: other bell peppers or pimentos, mushrooms, broccoli.
• May use other seasonings: ground or crushed red pepper, onion or garlic powder,
poultry seasoning.
• May sprinkle with parmesan cheese before serving.
Yield: 8 servings
Serving size: 1 cup

Barbecue Cups
Ingredients
¾ pounds lean ground turkey
½ cup spicy barbecue sauce*
2 teaspoons onion flakes dash garlic powder

1 10-ounces package low-fat refrigerator biscuits

Preparation Method
1. Brown turkey.
2. Add barbecue sauce, onion flakes, and garlic powder. Mix well.
3. Flatten each biscuit and press into muffin tin.
4. Spoon beef mixture into center of each biscuit cup.
5. Bake at 400°F for 10 to 12 minutes.

Nutritional content per serving
134 calories 0 grams trans fat 342 milligrams sodium 7 grams protein 27 milligrams cholesterol 151 milligrams potassium 5 grams total fat 13 grams carbohydrate 152-milligram phosphorus 1 grams saturated fat 0 grams fiber 11 milligrams calcium

Suggestions
• May use lean ground beef.
*Recipe included – see index.
Yield: 10 servings
Serving size: 1 biscuit

Seafood Croquettes
Ingredients
1 can water-packed salmon or tuna (14.75-ounce), or 1 pound frozen or fresh crab meat.
2 egg whites
¼ cup chopped onion
½ teaspoon black pepper
½ cup plain bread crumb or unsalted cracker crumbs
1 tablespoon vegetable oil or cooking spray
2 tablespoons lemon juice (optional)
½ teaspoon ground mustard (crab only)
¼ cup regular mayonnaise (tuna and crab only)

Preparation Method
1. Drain water from canned meat.
2. Combine all ingredients except oil in a medium bowl. Mix well.
3. Form mixture into 8 separate balls, and then flatten to form patties.

4. Heat vegetable oil in skillet.
5. Place patties in hot oil.
6. Brown patties on each side. If cooked in oil, drain patties on paper towel.

Nutritional content per serving
189 calories 0 grams trans fat 337 milligrams sodium 14 grams protein 81 milligrams cholesterol 184 milligrams potassium 8 grams total fat 11 grams carbohydrate 191 milligrams phosphorus 2 grams saturated fat 1 gram fibers 124 milligrams calcium

Suggestions
- May bake or broil patties in oven.
- May add chopped green pepper, celery, onion powder, garlic powder, Italian seasoning,

or curry powder.
Yield: 8 patties
Serving size: 1 patty

Baked Fish
Ingredients
4 3-ounce trout fillets or any other baking Fish
1 ½ teaspoon black pepper
1 tablespoon garlic powder
1 ½ teaspoon paprika
¼ medium green pepper
1 small onion
1 small lemon
2 tablespoons parmesan cheese

Preparation Method
1. Preheat oven to 375°F.
2. Place fish in a greased baking pan or on aluminum foil.
3. Sprinkle black pepper, garlic powder, and paprika on both sides of Fish.
4. Cut green peppers into strips and place on Fish. Slice onions into rings and place on Fish.
5. Squeeze juice of lemon onto Fish.
6. Bake for 30 minutes.

7. Afer Fish has cooked, sprinkle with parmesan cheese. Serve hot.

Nutritional content per serving

164 calories 0 grams trans fat 86 milligrams sodium 20 grams protein 62 milligrams cholesterol 452 milligrams potassium 6 grams fat 8 grams carbohydrate 252 milligrams phosphorus 1 grams saturated 3 grams fiber 80 milligrams calcium

Yield: 4 servings
Serving size: 3-ounces

Shrimp Salad
Ingredients
1 pound shrimp, boiled, chopped and deveined
1 hard-boiled egg, chopped
1 tablespoon celery, chopped
1 tablespoon green pepper, chopped
1 tablespoon onion, chopped
2 tablespoons mayonnaise
1 teaspoon lemon juice
½ teaspoon chili powder
⅛ teaspoon Tabasco® or hot sauce
½ teaspoon dry mustard lettuce, chopped or shredded (optional)

Preparation Method
1. Combine all ingredients except lettuce in a mixing bowl; mix well.
2. Chill in refrigerator for 30 minutes.
3. Serve as a salad over a bed of lettuce, if desired, or serve on a sandwich.

Nutritional content per serving

157 calories 0 grams trans fat 232 milligrams sodium 26 grams protein 234 milligrams cholesterol 233 milligrams potassium 5 grams total fat 1 gram carbohydrate 263 milligrams phosphorus 1 grams saturated fat 0 grams fiber 67 milligrams calcium

Suggestions
- May use frozen shrimp.
- May use scallops.

Yield: 4 servings

Serving size: ½ cup

Supreme of Seafood
Ingredients
1 cup crabmeat, cooked (boiled)
1 cup shrimp, cooked (boiled)
4 tablespoons green pepper, chopped
2 tablespoons green onions, chopped
1 cup celery, chopped
½ cup frozen green peas
½ teaspoon black pepper
½ cup mayonnaise
1 cup bread crumbs

Preparation Method
1. Preheat oven to 375°F.
2. Combine all ingredients except bread crumbs in a bowl.
3. Place in a greased casserole dish.
4. Top with bread crumbs.
5. Bake for 30 minutes.

Nutritional content per serving
220 calories 0 grams trans fat 445 milligrams sodium 16 grams protein 28 milligrams cholesterol 255 milligrams potassium 8 grams total fat 20 grams carbohydrate 148 milligrams phosphorus 1 grams saturated fat 2 grams fibers 85 milligrams calcium

Suggestions
- May use canned crabmeat, drain, and rinse.
- May use light mayonnaise.
- May use pepper of choice.

Yield: 6 servings
Serving size: ½ cup

Crab Cakes
Ingredients
1 egg (egg substitute or egg white optional)
⅓ cup green or red pepper, finely chopped
⅓ cup low sodium crackers

¼ cup reduced-fat mayonnaise
1 tablespoon dry mustard
1 teaspoon crushed red pepper or black pepper
2 tablespoons lemon juice
1 teaspoon garlic powder
2 tablespoon vegetable oil

Preparation Method
1. Combine all ingredients.
2. Divide into 6 balls and form patties.
3. Heat vegetable oil in pan at medium heat or oven at 350°F.
4. Fry patties 4-5 minutes or bake 15 minutes in oven.
5. Serve warm.

Nutritional content per serving
101 calories 0 grams trans fat 67 milligrams sodium 2 grams protein 41 milligrams cholesterol 72 milligrams potassium 9 grams total fat 5 grams carbohydrate 43 milligrams phosphorus 1 grams saturated fat 0 grams fibers 16 milligrams calcium
Yield: 6 servings
Serving size: 1 patty

Fish Tacos
Ingredients
12-16 Fish fillets (1 pound), tilapia or as desired
20 saltine crackers, unsalted tops, crushed finely
¼ cup unsalted butter or margarine
2 teaspoon dill weed
1 teaspoon garlic powder
¼ cup lemon juice

Preparation Method
1. Preheat oven to 400°F.
2. Combine crackers, garlic, and dill.
3. Melt butter or margarine.
4. Roll Fish in melted butter, then in crumbs and again in butter mix.
5. Place in baking pan and bake 8-10 minutes until Fish is flakey.

Nutritional content per serving
164 calories 0 grams trans fat 138 milligrams sodium 21 grams protein 57 milligrams cholesterol 335 milligrams potassium 6 grams total fat 7 grams carbohydrate 181 milligrams phosphorus 4 grams saturated fat 0 grams fibers 23 milligrams calcium

Suggestions
• Add to warmed tortillas.
• May top with sautéed onions, coleslaw, and fresh cilantro.
Yield: 4 servings
Serving size: 3 ½-ounces

Combination meals
This Set of meals can be combined with others of your choice to give an extra satisfaction.

Stuffed Green Peppers
Ingredients
2 tablespoon vegetable oil
½ pound ground lean beef, turkey or chicken
¼ cup onions, chopped
¼ cup celery, chopped
2 tablespoons lemon juice
1 tablespoon celery seed
2 tablespoons Italian seasoning
1 teaspoon black pepper
½ teaspoon sugar
1 ½ cups cooked rice
6 small green peppers, seeded with tops removed paprika

Preparation Method
1. Preheat oven to 325°F.
2. Heat oil in saucepan.
3. Add ground meat, onions, and celery, cook until meat is browned.
4. Add all ingredients except green peppers and paprika to saucepan. Stir together, remove from heat.
5. Stuff peppers with mixture. Wrap with foil or place in a dish and cover. Bake for 30 minutes. Remove and sprinkle with

paprika.

Nutritional content per serving
131 calories 0 grams trans fat 36 milligrams sodium 9 grams protein 28 milligrams cholesterol 160 milligrams potassium 4 grams total fat 15 grams carbohydrate 83 milligrams phosphorus 1 gram saturated fat 1 gram fibers 38 milligrams calcium
Yield: 6 servings
Serving size: 1 stuffed pepper

Rotini with Mock Italian Sausage
Ingredients
4 ounces uncooked rotini pasta
¾ pound lean ground turkey
1 cup onion, chopped
1 clove garlic, minced
½ cup chopped celery
¾ teaspoon Italian seasoning
¼ teaspoon fennel seeds
¼ teaspoon crushed red pepper
3 tablespoons tomato paste
1-14 ½ unsalted can (190 grams) tomatoes, chopped
2 tablespoons grated parmesan cheese

Preparation Method
1. Boil rotini pasta according to package directions, drain.
2. Sauté turkey in a non-stick skillet over medium heat until browned, stirring to crumble. Drain on paper towel.
3. Add onion, garlic, celery, and seasonings. Cook 3 minutes, stirring occasionally.
4. Add tomato paste and tomatoes. Partially cover, reduce heat, and simmer 15 minutes.
5. Serve over rotini. Top with cheese.

Nutritional content per serving
165 calories 0 grams trans fat 250 milligrams sodium 13 grams protein 41 milligrams cholesterol 458 milligrams potassium 2 grams total fat 28 grams carbohydrate 161 milligrams phosphorus 1 grams saturated fat 2 grams fibers 65 milligrams calcium

Main dishes
Yield: 4 servings
Serving size: ¾ cups turkey mixture and 1 cup rotini

Eggplant Casserole
Ingredients
1 large eggplant
2 tablespoon vegetable oil
½ cup green pepper, chopped
½ cup onion, finely chopped
1 pound lean ground beef or turkey
2 cups plain bread crumbs
1 large egg, slightly beaten
½ teaspoon red pepper, optional

Preparation Method
1. Preheat oven to 350°F.
2. Boil eggplant until tender; drain and mash.
3. Heat oil; add green pepper, onion, and ground meat. Sauté until cooked.
4. Add eggplant, bread crumbs, and egg, mixing well.
5. Add red pepper to taste, if desired.
6. Bake in casserole dish for 30-45 minutes. Serve warm.

Nutritional content per serving
240 calories 0 grams trans fat 263 milligrams sodium 15 grams protein 74 milligrams cholesterol 380 milligrams potassium 9 grams total fat 5 grams carbohydrate 169 milligrams phosphorus 2 grams saturated fat 4 grams fibers 71 milligrams calcium
Yield: 8 servings
Serving size: ½ cup

Stir Fry Meal
Ingredients
2 tablespoon cooking oil
2 medium chicken breast, cut in bite-size pieces
1 10-ounce package frozen stir fry vegetables
½ tablespoon low sodium soy sauce
2 cups cooked rice

Preparation Method
1. Heat oil in 9-10" skillet on high.
2. Add chicken, and sauté.
3. Stir in vegetables.
4. Add soy sauce and stir well.
5. Reduce heat to medium-high and cook uncovered for 3-5 minutes, or until done, stirring frequently.
6. Serve over ⅔ cup rice.

Nutritional content per serving
315 calories 0 grams trans fat 37 milligrams sodium 29 grams protein 76 milligrams cholesterol 618 milligrams potassium 7 grams total fat 32 grams carbohydrate 26 milligrams phosphorus 2 grams saturated fat 3 grams fibers 32 milligrams calcium

Suggestion
• May use 6-ounces of shrimp instead of chicken.
Yield: 3 servings
Serving size: ½ cup chicken and vegetables with ⅔ cup rice

New Orleans-Style Rice Dressing
Ingredients
2 tablespoons vegetable oil ¼ cup green peppers, chopped
1 pound lean ground turkey ½ teaspoon cayenne pepper
2 tablespoons all-purpose flour 1 clove garlic, chopped
¼ cup onion, chopped 2 cups hot cooked rice
¼ cup green onions, chopped 1 cup low sodium chicken broth
¼ cup celery, chopped

Preparation Method
1. Heat oven to 350°F.
2. Heat oil in skillet, add meat and cook on medium heat until browned.
3. Remove meat and drain on paper towel.
4. Add flour to skillet and brown to make a dark roux.
5. Add onions, celery, peppers, and garlic to roux and cook until vegetables are tender.
6. Add cooked rice and meat to skillet.

7. Add low sodium broth a little at a time until mixture is moist. If mixture is too dry may add water.
8. Pour into a 1 ½ quart baking dish.
9. Bake for 20 minutes

Nutritional content per serving
393 calories 0 grams trans fat 113 milligrams sodium 27 grams protein 84 milligrams cholesterol 377 milligrams potassium 19 grams total fat 28 grams carbohydrate 228 milligrams phosphorus 4 grams saturated 1 grams fibers 43 milligrams calcium

Suggestions
• Substitute lean beef with lean turkey.
Yield: 4 servings
Serving size: 1 cup

Fajitas
Ingredients
2 tablespoon vegetable oil
1 ½ pounds raw chicken strips or beef strips or shrimp (peeled and deveined)
2 teaspoon chili powder
½ teaspoon cumin
2 tablespoon lemon or lime juice
¼ green and/or red pepper, sliced lengthwise
½ onion white, sliced lengthwise
½ teaspoon dry cilantro
4 flour tortillas
vegetable spray

Preparation Method
1. Preheat oven to 300°F.
2. Add vegetable oil to non-stick frying pan over medium heat.
3. Add meat, seasonings, and lemon/lime juice; cook for 5-10 minutes or until tender.
4. Add pepper and onion to pan and cook 1-2 minutes.
5. Remove from heat; add cilantro.
6. Place tortillas on foil and move to oven. Heat for 10 minutes
7. Divide mixture between tortillas, wrap, and serve.

Nutritional content per serving
184 calories 0 grams trans fat 121 milligrams sodium 19 grams protein 57 milligrams cholesterol 494 milligrams potassium 10 grams total fat 5 grams carbohydrates 207 milligrams phosphorus 1 gram saturated fat 1 gram fibers 38 milligrams calcium

Suggestions
• May use 1 tablespoon sour cream, ranch dressing or salsa.
• May serve over hot rice.
Yield: 4 servings
Serving size: 4 medium strips

Beef & Vegetable Soup
Ingredients
1 pound beef stew 3 ½ cups water
1 cup raw sliced onions ½ cup frozen green peas
1 teaspoon black pepper ½ cup frozen okra
½ teaspoon basil ½ cup frozen carrots, diced
½ teaspoon thyme ½ cup frozen corn

Preparation Method
1. 1. In a large pot, place beef stew, onions, black pepper, basil, thyme, and water. Cook for about 45 minutes.
2. Add all frozen vegetables; simmer on low heat until meat is tender. Serve hot.
3. Note: soup may require additional water. Add water ½ cup at a time as necessary.

Nutritional content per serving
190 calories 0 grams trans fat 56 milligrams sodium 11 grams protein 42 milligrams cholesterol 291 milligrams potassium 13 grams total fat 7 grams carbohydrates 121 milligrams phosphorus 5 grams saturated fat 2 grams fibers 31 milligrams calcium

Suggestions
• Other lower potassium vegetables may be used—green beans, cabbage, green peppers,
  celery, yellow squash. Noodles may also be added.
• Other seasonings that may be used: salt-free bouillon cubes,

marjoram, onion powder, garlic powder, Italian seasoning, curry powder, bay leaf.

Reminder: soup must be counted as part of daily fluid allowance.

Yield: 8 servings

Serving size: ¾ cup

Great Soup recipes Chicken Noodle Soup
Ingredients

1 pound chicken parts 1 teaspoon red pepper
¼ cup lemon juice 1 teaspoon caraway seed
3 ½ cups water 1 teaspoon oregano
1 tablespoon poultry seasoning 1 teaspoon sugar
1 teaspoon garlic powder ½ cup celery
1 teaspoon onion powder ½ cup green pepper
2 tablespoons vegetable oil 1 cup egg noodles
1 teaspoon black pepper

Preparation Method

1. Rub chicken parts with lemon juice.
2. In a large pot, combine chicken, water, poultry seasoning, garlic powder, onion powder, vegetable oil, black pepper, red pepper, caraway seed, oregano, and sugar together. Cook 30 minutes or until chicken is tender.
3. Add remaining ingredients and cook for an additional 15 minutes. Serve hot.

Note: Soup may require additional water; if so, add water ½ cup at a time.

Nutritional content per serving

110 calories 0 grams trans fat 17 milligrams sodium 3 grams protein 12 milligrams cholesterol 101 milligrams potassium 8 grams fat 7 grams carbohydrate 39 milligrams phosphorus 2 grams saturated 0 grams fibers 21 milligrams calcium

Yield: 8 servings

Serving size: ¾ cup

Soups

Suggestions

- Other vegetables may be used: onions, mushrooms, carrots, pimentos, green peas, green beans, or whole kernel corn.
- Additional seasonings that may be used are sage, rosemary, marjoram, thyme, bay leaf, basil, and dill seed.
- May use whole boneless chicken parts, without skin
- May be served with unsalted crackers or regular bread.

Reminder: count soup as part of daily fluid allowance.

Herbed Omelet
Ingredients
1 ½ teaspoons vegetable oil
1 tablespoon chopped onion
4 eggs
2 tablespoons water
¼ teaspoon basil
⅛ teaspoon tarragon
¼ teaspoon parsley (optional)

Preparation Method
1. Beat eggs; add water and spices.
2. Heat oil in 8" frying pan over medium heat, add onions and sauté. Remove from pan.
3. Pour mixture into heated frying pan over medium heat.
4. As the omelet sets, lif with a spatula to let the uncooked portion of the omelet flow to the bottom.
5. When the omelet is completely set, add the sautéed onion to the top of the omelet and remove from pan to a serving dish.

Nutritional content per serving
195 calories 0 grams trans fat 157 milligrams sodium 14 grams protein 474 milligrams cholesterol 157 milligrams potassium 15-gram total fat 0 grams carbohydrate 214 milligrams phosphorus 4 grams saturated fat 0 grams fibers 60 milligrams calcium

Suggestions
- May include bell pepper.
- May use egg substitutes or egg whites in place of whole eggs.

Yield: 2 servings
Serving size: ½ omelet

Egg Dishes Fruit Omelet
Ingredients
2 cups frozen unsweetened strawberries, thawed
1 tablespoon sugar (optional)
4 eggs, separated
1 tablespoon lemon juice
1 tablespoon unsalted butter or margarine

Preparation Method
1. Preheat oven to 375°F.
2. Sprinkle thawed strawberries with sugar; let stand.
3. Beat egg whites in a medium bowl until stiff.
4. Beat egg yolks and lemon juice in a separate bowl. Fold stiffly beaten egg whites into beaten yolks until no yellow streaks remain.
5. Melt butter in a 10" skillet that is oven-safe. Pour egg mixture into skillet, tilting pan to coat sides. Cook over low heat 5 minutes.
6. When mixture is set on the bottom, cook in oven for 5 additional minutes.
7. Lif omelet onto heated plate. Spoon on strawberries. Cut into pie wedges. Serve hot.

Nutritional content per serving
198 calories 0 grams trans fat 125 milligrams sodium 8 grams protein 240 milligrams cholesterol 430 milligrams potassium 9 grams total fat 24 grams carbohydrate 141 milligrams phosphorus 4 grams saturated fat 7 grams fibers 56 milligrams calcium

Suggestions
• Other fruits may be substituted: dutch apples, cherries, blueberries, blackberries,   or   canned peaches.
• Spices that may be included: allspice, cinnamon, or nutmeg.
Yield: 4 servings
Serving size: ¼ omelet

Baking Powder Biscuits
Ingredients
2 cups all-purpose flour, sifted
3 teaspoons double-acting baking powder
2 teaspoons sugar
⅓ cup vegetable shortening
¼ cup 1% milk
½ cup water

Preparation Method
1. Pre-heat oven at 350°F.
1. Sif dry ingredients into a bowl.
2. Cut in shortening until coarse crumbs form. Make a well in the mixture.
3. Pour milk and water into the well.
4. Stir quickly with a fork until dough follows fork around the bowl.
5. Dough should be soft. Turn dough onto lightly floured surface.
6. Knead gently 10-12 times. Roll or pat dough until ½" thick.
7. Dip a 2 ½" biscuit cutter into flour; then cut out 10 biscuits.
8. Bake biscuits on ungreased baking sheet for 12-15 minutes.

Nutritional content per serving
162 calories 1 gram trans fat 150 milligrams sodium 3 grams protein 1 milligrams cholesterol 36 milligrams potassium 8 grams total fat 21 grams carbohydrate 63 milligrams phosphorus 2 grams saturated fat 1 gram fibers 92 milligrams calcium
Yield: 10 biscuits
Serving size: 1 biscuit

Old Fashioned Pancakes
Ingredients
½ cup all-purpose flour
1 egg, beaten
¼ cup granulated sugar
¼ teaspoon baking powder
¼ cup 2% milk plus ¼ cup water
1 tablespoon vegetable oil

Preparation Method

1. Combine first four ingredients in a bowl. Mix well. Add milk and water. Add more water for thinner pancakes or less for thicker pancakes.
2. Heat oil in a skillet or on a griddle. Pour ¼ cup batter on griddle. Cook until brown, turning on each side.

Nutritional content per serving

165 calories 0 grams trans fat 58 milligrams sodium 4 grams protein 61 milligrams cholesterol 57 milligrams potassium 5 grams total fat 26 grams carbohydrates 64 milligrams phosphorus 1 gram saturated 0 grams fibers 45 milligram calcium

Yield: 4 small pancakes
Serving size: 1 pancake

French Toast
Ingredients
4 large egg whites, slightly beaten
¼ cup 1% milk
½ teaspoon cinnamon
¼ teaspoon allspice
4 slices white bread (maybe toasted)
1 tablespoon margarine

Preparation Method
1. Add milk, cinnamon, and allspice to egg whites.
2. Dip bread into batter one piece at a time.
3. Place on heated grill or in skillet with melted margarine.
4. Turn bread after it is golden brown.
5. Serve hot with syrup (sugar-free if diabetic).

Nutritional content per serving

125 calories 0 grams trans fat 194 milligrams sodium 7 grams protein 0 milligrams cholesterol 128 milligrams potassium 5 grams total fat 14 grams carbohydrate 61 milligrams phosphorus 0 grams saturated fat 1 gram fibers 60 milligrams calcium

Suggestions
• May add ½ cup egg substitute.
Yield: 4 servings

Serving size: 1 slice

White Bread Dressing
Ingredients
2 tablespoons margarine
¼ cup chopped onions
1 ½ cups plain bread crumbs or 3 slices bread, crumbled
¼ cup chopped celery
1 teaspoon poultry seasoning
¼ teaspoon garlic powder
¼ cup unsalted chicken broth

Preparation Method
1. Melt margarine in a small skillet. Add onions. Stir until onions are tender.
2. Add bread crumbs, stirring constantly to prevent scorching.
3. Remove from heat. Add celery, poultry seasoning, garlic powder, and chicken broth.
4. Blend well. Place in a small baking pan.
5. Bake for 30 minutes at 375°F.
6. If dressing appears too dry, add water as needed.

Nutritional content per serving
107 calories 0 grams trans fat 129 milligrams sodium 2 grams protein 11 grams carbohydrates 77 milligrams potassium 6 grams total fat 11 milligrams cholesterol 30 milligrams phosphorus 0 grams saturated 1 gram fibers 35 milligrams calcium

Suggestions
- May use homemade broth made from cooked chicken.
- Uncooked dressing will keep for 1-2 months in freezer.
- Additional breadcrumbs may be added.
- If a small iron skillet is used, the dressing may be baked in the skillet.

Yield: 4 servings
Serving size: ½ cup

Cornbread Dressing
Yield: 15 servings

Serving size: 2" x 2" square or ¾ cup

Directions for cornbread
1. Preheat oven to 425°F.
2. Combine cornmeal, flour, sugar, and baking powder in mixing bowl; mix well.
3. Add water, egg, and oil, mixing well.
4. Place in a 9" x 9" square greased baking pan.
5. Bake until golden brown.
6. When done, let cool, then crumble. Set aside to combine with dressing ingredients.

Ingredients for cornbread
2 cups cornmeal (plain)
1 ½ cups all-purpose flour
2 ½ cups water
1 egg
2 tablespoons vegetable oil

Ingredients for dressing
2 cups chicken parts and giblets
4 cups water
1 cup chopped onion
½ cup chopped celery
½ cup chopped green peppers
1 teaspoon black pepper
1 teaspoon poultry seasoning
1 teaspoon onion powder
1 teaspoon sage

Directions for dressing
1. 1. Wash chicken parts and giblets and add to water in a large pot.
2. Add onion, celery, green pepper and black pepper.
3. Boil for 30 minutes until tender
4. When done, reserve 2 cups of broth for dressing (remaining broth may be used for giblet gravy on the following page). Let meat cool.
5. Remove meat from bone and add to remaining dressing

ingredients.
6. Mix all ingredients together with 2 cups broth from chicken until mixture is moist.
7. Spread into baking pan.
8. Bake at 425°F until golden brown.

Nutritional content per serving

156 calories 0 grams trans fat 75 milligrams sodium 4 grams protein 16 milligrams cholesterol 88 milligrams potassium 3 grams total fat 29 grams carbohydrate 62 milligrams phosphorus 0 grams saturated 2 grams fibers 48 milligrams calcium

Suggestions
• May substitute turkey parts and giblets for chicken. Cornbread Dressing

Giblet Gravy
Ingredients
2 cups chicken broth (homemade from boiled chicken)
1 tablespoon all-purpose flour
1 hard-boiled egg, sliced or chopped
1-2 poultry liver or giblets, boiled, chopped

Preparation Method
1. Stir 1 tablespoon of broth with flour until smooth.
2. Add remaining broth and cook over low heat, stirring constantly.
3. Add boiled egg and giblets.
4. Continue to stir until desired thickness (about 5 minutes).

Nutritional content per serving

13 calories 0 grams trans fat 13 milligrams sodium 1 gram protein 13 milligrams cholesterol 31 milligrams potassium 0 grams total fat 1 gram carbohydrate 16 milligrams phosphorus 0 grams saturated fat 0 grams fibers 3 milligrams calcium

Suggestions
• Use on your favorite dressing or vegetable.
Yield: 32 servings
Serving size: 1 tablespoon

Corn Pudding
Ingredients
2 cups kernel corn, canned or fresh cut
3 slightly beaten eggs or ¾ cup egg substitute
½ cup 1% milk
½ cup water
⅓ cup onion, finely chopped
1 tablespoon butter, melted
1 teaspoon granulated sugar
1 teaspoon white or black pepper

Preparation Method
1. Preheat oven to 350°F.
2. Combine all ingredients.
3. Pour into a greased 1 ½-quart casserole dish.
4. Place in a shallow pan filled with 1 inch of hot water.
5. Bake 40-45 minutes, or until knife inserted in center comes out clean.
6. Let stand for 10 minutes at room temperature before serving.

Nutritional content per serving
120 calories 0 grams trans fat 61 milligrams sodium 6 grams protein 121 milligrams cholesterol 234 milligrams potassium 5 grams total fat 17 grams carbohydrate 122 milligrams phosphorus 2.0 grams saturated 2 grams fibers 49 milligrams calcium
Yield: 6 servings
Serving size: ½ cup

Herb Rice Casserole
Ingredients
1 cup white rice, uncooked
2 cups chicken stock, unsalted
¼ cup green bell pepper, chopped
½ teaspoon parsley flakes
1 tablespoon vegetable oil
3 Fresh green onions, chopped
1 tablespoon chives

Preparation Method
1. Preheat oven to 350°F.
2. Combine all ingredients, and place in casserole dish.
3. Bake in covered casserole for 45-50 minutes or until liquid is absorbed.

Nutritional content per serving
53 calories 0 grams trans fat 19 milligrams sodium 2 grams protein 7 grams carbohydrate 74 milligrams potassium 2 grams total fat 0 milligrams cholesterol 29 milligrams phosphorus 0 saturated 0 grams fibers 7 milligrams calcium

Suggestions
• Serve with your favorite chicken dish and vegetable.
Yield: 8 servings
Serving size: ½ cup

Yeast Dinner Rolls
Ingredients
1 cup hot water
6 tablespoons vegetable shortening
½ cup sugar
1 package yeast
2 tablespoons of warm water
1 egg
3 ¾-4 cups all-purpose flour

Preparation Method
1. Preheat oven to 400°F.
2. Combine hot water, shortening, and sugar in a large bowl. Set aside to cool to room temperature.
3. Dissolve yeast in warm water.
4. Add egg, yeast, and half the flour to the mixture in the large bowl. Beat well.
5. Stir in the remaining flour with a spoon until easy to handle.
6. Place dough in a greased bowl; grease top and cover top with plastic wrap.
7. Allow to rest 1 to 1 ½ hours or until the dough has doubled in size.

8. Cut off amount needed to shape rolls.
9. Bake rolls for 12 minutes or until done.

Nutritional content per serving
148 calories 0 grams trans fat 5 milligrams sodium 3 grams protein 12 milligrams cholesterol 31 milligrams potassium 4 grams total fat 24 grams carbohydrate 32 milligrams phosphorus 1 grams saturated 1 gram fibers 5 milligrams calcium

Suggestions
- Use for all occasions: breakfast, lunch, dinner, and homemade bread.

Yield: 20 servings
Serving size: 1 roll

Blueberry Muffins
Ingredients
1 egg white
¼ cup margarine
½ cup sugar
7 tablespoons water
½ teaspoon vanilla extract
1 teaspoon baking powder
1 cup all-purpose flour
1 cup blueberries, canned and drained or fresh

Preparation Method
1. Preheat oven to 375°F.
2. Beat egg white in a small mixing bowl until stiff. Set aside.
3. Cream margarine and sugar together until smooth.
4. Add water and vanilla, mixing thoroughly.
5. Add baking powder and flour.
6. Fold in beaten egg white and blueberries.
7. Bake in greased muffin pan for 30 minutes.

Nutritional content per serving
123 calories 0 grams trans fat 139 milligrams sodium 1.5 grams protein 0 milligrams cholesterol 71 milligrams potassium 4 grams total fat 21 grams carbohydrate 94 milligrams phosphorus

0 saturated fat 1 gram fibers 29 milligrams calcium

Suggestions
- May use strawberries, blackberries, or raspberries instead of blueberries.

Yield: 12 muffins
Serving size: 1 muffin

Blueberry Baked Bread
Ingredients
1 quart blueberries, fresh or frozen
¼ cup water (omit if berries are frozen)
1 teaspoon lemon juice
½ cup sugar
1 pinch nutmeg
1 pinch cinnamon
1 tablespoon margarine
3 slices bread, buttered and sprinkled with cinnamon and sugar on both sides

Preparation Method
1. Heat oven to 425°F.
2. Wash blueberries under cool running water.
3. Combine all ingredients in a saucepan except bread. Bring to a boil.
4. Pour blueberry mixture into a shallow baking pan; top with bread cut in halves.
5. Bake until brown (about 10 minutes).

Nutritional content per serving
176 calories 0 grams trans fat 92 milligrams sodium 2 grams protein 0 milligrams cholesterol 83 milligrams potassium 3 grams total fat 39 grams carbohydrate 20 milligrams phosphorus 0 saturated fat 3 grams fibers 56 milligrams calcium

Suggestions
- May be used as dessert or snack.
- Other fruits may also be used: strawberries, cherries, apples, blackberries, or canned peaches.

- To enhance the flavor of the fruit may use allspice or brown sugar.

Yield: 6 servings
Serving size: ½ cup

Herb Bread
Ingredients
1 loaf french bread
¼ cup margarine (unsalted)
2 tablespoons chopped green onions
1 teaspoon thyme
¼ teaspoon tarragon
1 teaspoon basil flakes (optional)
½ teaspoon crushed marjoram (optional)

Preparation Method
1. Heat oven to 350°F.
2. Slice french bread almost to the bottom crust.
3. Combine margarine with remaining ingredients.
4. Spread butter mixture on cut surfaces or slices. May use a brush.

5. Place on a baking sheet or pan.
6. Bake for 15-20 minutes.

Nutritional content per serving
120 calories 0 grams trans fat 208 milligrams sodium 4 grams protein 44 milligrams potassium 0 milligrams cholesterol 4 grams total fat 18 grams carbohydrate 37 milligrams phosphorus 1 grams saturated fat 1 grams fibers 15 milligrams calcium

Suggestions
- May omit spices and substitute with 2 teaspoons parsley flakes.

Yield: 1 loaf — about 15 slice
Serving size: 1 slice

CHAPTER IV: Food to avoid for a healthy kidney

It is well-known life is full of do's and don'ts, thus we would consider common food one should avoid in order to live a healthy life.

The Causes of kidney failure are numerous. The most widely recognized are hypertension which is also known as High blood pressure and diabetes (in an uncontrolled state).

Liquor addiction, coronary illness, hepatitis C infection, and HIV contamination are likewise causes.

At the point when the kidneys become damaged and can't work appropriately, liquid can develop in the body, and waste can amass in the blood.

Regardless, evading or restricting certain nourishments that are part of your eating menu may help decline the aggregation of waste items in the blood, improve kidney work, and avoid further harm.

Dietary restrictions change based upon the phase of kidney sickness. For example, individuals who are in the beginning periods of incessant kidney infection will have unexpected dietary limitations in comparison to those with end-arrange renal sickness or kidney disappointment.

Those with end-stage renal ailment who require dialysis will likewise have changing dietary limitations. Dialysis is a sort of treatment that evacuates additional water and channels waste.

Most of those in the late stages or with end-stage kidney ailment should pursue a kidney-accommodating diet to evade develop of specific synthetic substances or supplements in the blood.

In those with constant kidney illness, the kidneys can't sufficiently evacuate abundance sodium, potassium, and phosphorus. Accordingly, they are at higher danger of increased blood levels of these minerals.

A kidney-accommodating diet, or a "renal diet," generally incorporates restricting sodium and potassium to 2,000 milligrams for each day and constraining phosphorus to 1,000 milligrams for every day.
Damaged kidneys may likewise experience difficulty sifting the waste results of protein digestion. In this way, people with incessant kidney disease in stages 1–4 may need to restrict the measure of protein in their weight control plans.

In anyway, those with end-organize renal ailment experiencing dialysis have an expanded protein prerequisite.

Here is a list of 20 foods that if possible, should be completely avoided, or if not, should be seldom eaten.

1. Dark-Colored Colas
Despite the calories that colas relinquish, they in like manner contain substances that include phosphorus, especially in dark colas.

Various sustenance makers incorporate phosphorus during the treatment of food and beverages to improve season, draw out time allotment of sensible ease of use, and prevent recoloring.

This additional phosphorus is considerably more absorbable by the human body than regular, creature, or plant-based phosphorus.

In contrast to regular phosphorus, phosphorus as added substances isn't bound to protein. Or maybe, it's found as salt and profoundly absorbable by the intestinal tract.

Added substance phosphorus can normally be found in an item's fixing rundown. Regardless, nourishment makers are not required to list the definite measure of added substance phosphorus on the nourishment mark.

While added substance phosphorus content shifts relying upon the sort of cola, most dull hued colas are accepted to contain 50–100 milligrams in a 200-ml serving.

Subsequently, colas, particularly those dull in shading, ought to be stayed away from on a renal eating routine.

2. Avocados

Avocados are regularly touted for their numerous nutritious characteristics, including their heart-solid fats, fiber, and cell reinforcements.

While avocados are generally a solid expansion to the eating regimen, people with kidney ailment may have to avoid them, if they are to continue to enjoy good health.

This is on the grounds that avocados are an extremely rich wellspring of potassium. One cup (150 grams) of avocado gives an astounding 727 milligrams of potassium.

That is twofold the measure of potassium than a medium banana gives. Along these lines, avocados, including guacamole, ought to be kept away in relation with a renal diet menu, particularly if perhaps you have been advised to watch your potassium intake.

3. Canned Foods

Canned nourishment, for example, soups, vegetables, and beans are frequently obtained due to their minimal effort and comfort.

In any case, most canned nourishments contain high measures of sodium, as salt is added as an additive to expand its timeframe of realistic usability.

Due to the measure of sodium found in canned merchandise, it's frequently prescribed that individuals with kidney ailment dodge or breaking point their utilization.

Picking lower-sodium assortments or those named "no salt included" is ordinarily best. Furthermore, depleting and washing canned nourishments, such as canned beans and fish, can diminish the sodium content by 33–80%, contingent upon the item.

4. Whole-Wheat Bread

Picking the right bread can be mistaking for people with kidney disease. Regularly for sound people, entire wheat bread is normally prescribed over refined, white flour bread.

Entire wheat bread might be an increasingly nutritious decision, for the most part, this is due to the content of fiber that is contained in high quantity. So therefore, white bread is typically prescribed over entire wheat assortments for people with kidney illness.

Note that most bread and bread items, paying little heed to being white or entire wheat, additionally contain moderately high measures of sodium.

It's ideal to look at sustenance names of different kinds of bread, pick a lower-sodium alternative, if conceivable, and screen your bit sizes.

5. Brown Rice

Like entire wheat bread, darker rice is an entire grain that has a much larger content of phosphorus and potassium than its white counterpart.

145-150 milligrams of phosphorus and 150-154 milligrams of potassium is readily contained in a full cup of dark colored cooked rice, compared to its white colored counterpart that contains about 65-60 milligrams and 50-54 milligrams of potassium.

While it is possible to fit in dark-colored rice when following a renal diet menu, there would have to then be a controlling and offsetting with different nourishments to keep away from exorbitant day by day admission of these minerals.

Bulgur, buckwheat, pearled grain, and couscous are nutritious, lower-phosphorus grains that can make a decent substitute for darker rice.

6. Bananas

Bananas have a high level of potassium and this one of its outstanding benefits, but not to renal patients. They are relatively low in sodium; one fair-sized banana gives about 442 milligrams of potassium.

Knowing this, the possibility of keeping your potassium level intake to 2,000 milligrams would be quite challenging, if bananas are a regular part of your day to day diet.

Lamentably, numerous other tropical natural products have high potassium substance too. Either way, pineapples contain significantly less potassium than other tropical leafy foods be a progressively reasonable, yet delectable, elective.

Rundown Bananas are a rich wellspring of potassium and may should be restricted on a renal eating routine. Pineapple is a kidney-accommodating organic product, as it contains considerably less potassium than certain other tropical natural products.

7. Dairy

Dairy items are rich in different vitamins and supplements. They're likewise a characteristic wellspring of phosphorus and potassium and a decent wellspring of protein.

For instance, 1 cup (8 liquid ounces) of entire milk contains about 345-349 milligrams of phosphorus and 220-222 milligrams of potassium.

However, if your consumption of dairy is excessive, related to different phosphorus-rich nourishments, can be unfavorable to bone wellbeing in those with kidney infection.

This may sound astonishing, as milk and dairy are regularly suggested for solid bones and muscle wellbeing. In this regard, when the kidneys are harmed, a lot of phosphorus utilization can cause a development of phosphorus in the blood. This can make your bones slim and feeble after some time and expand the danger of bone breakage or crack.

Dairy items are likewise high in protein. One cup (8 liquid ounces) of entire milk gives around 8 grams of protein. It might be imperative to restrict dairy admission to stay away from the development of protein squander in the blood.

Dairy choices like unenriched rice milk and almond milk are a lot of lower in potassium, phosphorus, and protein than bovine's milk, making them a decent substitute for milk while on a renal eating routine.

8. Oranges and Orange Juice
While oranges and squeezed orange are seemingly most outstanding for their nutrient C substance, they are likewise rich wellsprings of potassium.

One huge orange weighing about 180 - 184 grams gives approximately 330 - 333 milligrams of potassium. Given their potassium substance, oranges and squeezed orange likely should be kept away from or constrained on a renal eating regimen.

Grapes, apples, and cranberries, just as their particular juices, are on the whole great substitutes for oranges and squeezed orange, as they have lower potassium substance.

9. Processed Meats
Processed meats have, for some time, been related with incessant infections and are commonly viewed as unfortunate because of their substance of additives.

Processed meats will be meats that have been salted, dried, relieved, or canned. A few models incorporate wieners, bacon, pepperoni, jerky, and frankfurter.

Processed meats ordinarily contain quite a large amount of salt content, generally to improve taste and protect season.

In this manner, it might be hard to keep your day by day sodium admission to under 2,000 milligrams whenever processed meats are bounteous in your eating routine. Moreover, prepared meats are high in protein.

In the event that you have been advised to screen your protein admission, it's essential to confine prepared meats hence also.

10. Pickles, Olives, and Relish

Pickles, prepared olives and relish are on the whole instances of restored or salted nourishments. Typically, a lot of salt are included during the relieving or pickling process. For instance, one pickle lance can contain in excess of 300 milligrams of sodium. Similarly, there are 244 milligrams of sodium in 2 tablespoons of sweet pickle relish.

Numerous markets stock diminished sodium assortments of pickles, olives, and relish, which contain less sodium than the conventional assortments.

Regardless, even decreased sodium alternatives can at present be high in sodium, so you will, in any case, need to watch your parts.

In summary, Pickles, handled, olives and relish are high in sodium and ought to be constrained on a renal eating regimen.

11. Apricots

Apricots are high in potassium and rich in Fiber including vitamin A and C. One cup of crisp apricots gives 427 milligrams of potassium. Besides, the potassium content is much increasingly moved in dried apricots. One cup of dried apricots gives more than 1,500 milligrams of potassium.

This implies only one cup of dried apricots gives 75% of the 2,000 milligrams low-potassium confinement. When on a renal diet, it is advisable to keep apricots, especially the dry ones at arm's length.

12. Potatoes
Potatoes are potassium-rich vegetables, sweet potatoes inclusive. Only one medium-sized potato well prepared. contains potassium content up to 610, though one normal estimated heated sweet potato contains potassium content up to 541 milligrams

Luckily, some high-potassium nourishments like the aforementioned, when drenched or filtered can lessen their mineral content.

Cutting potatoes into little, slim pieces and bubbling them for in any event 10 minutes can diminish the potassium content by about half.

Potatoes that are absorbed an enormous pot of water for in any event four hours before cooking are demonstrated to have an even lower potassium content than those not doused before cooking. This strategy is known as "potassium draining," or the "twofold cook technique."

Albeit twofold cooking potatoes brings down the potassium content, it's imperative to recollect that their potassium content isn't finished dispensed with by this strategy. Impressive measures of potassium can even now be available in twofold cooked potatoes, so it's ideal to rehearse divide control to hold potassium levels under tight restraints.

13. Soda
Steer clear! Soft drink gives no nourishing advantage and is pressed with sugars - either normal or artificially produced. This likens to additional calories in your eating routine and can at last outcome in undesirable weight gain. A run of the mill 12 oz. cola has 152 calories, and in certain spots, this is viewed as a little serving of pop! Studies carried out have connected the effect of soft drinks to health conditions like metabolic disorder, kidney sickness, and dental issues. Diet soft drinks might be lower in calories, yet at the same time give no health benefit and frequently contain added substances, including counterfeit sugars. Skirt the pop and reach for water. In the event that you don't care for the flavor of plain water, include a cut or two of new

natural product to include enhance.

14. Butter

Skimp on the spread! Margarine is produced using creature fat and contains cholesterol, calories, and elevated levels of soaked fat. Margarine is produced using vegetable oil and is higher in the "great" fats, yet may not be a superior decision since it regularly contains trans fats. Whenever the situation allows, use canola or olive oil. For instance, that you choose a spread, go for one that is lower in calories and immersed fat and contains no trans fats.

15. Mayonnaise

Its mind bulging to know that over 102 calories is contained in one full tablespoon of mayonnaise! In addition to the fact that its calorie content is way above normal, it also contains high level of immersed fat. Lower calorie and without fat mayonnaise are accessible available, yet they regularly contain a high amount of sugar content as well as that of sodium and may also contain other added substances. A more beneficial swap includes supplanting your mayonnaise with plain non-fat Greek yogurt, which is high in protein and blends pleasantly to tie servings of mixed greens.

16. Frozen foods

Studies have indicated that processed nourishments may add to the advancement of type 2 diabetes, and solidified or pre-made dinners like solidified pizza and microwaveable meals are regularly intensely prepared. Substantial preparing can mean concealed sugar, sodium, and fat. Regardless, not every single solidified supper is made equivalent! It is constantly a smart thought to get ready new nourishments when you can, however, if that comfort is critical, perhaps that you pick solidified dinners, read the names cautiously. Search for those that are "low sodium" or "no sodium included" and stay away from solidified suppers with included sugar, fillers, or some other added substances. Parity out the dinner by including crisp foods grown from the ground in the event that they are excluded from the solidified feast.

17. Tomatoes

Tomatoes are another high-potassium organic product that may not fit the rules of a renal eating regimen. They can be served crude or stewed and are regularly used to make sauces. Only one cup of tomato sauce can contain as much as 900 milligrams of potassium.

Tragically for those on a renal eating regimen, tomatoes are normally utilized in numerous dishes. Picking an option with lower potassium content depends generally on taste inclination. In any case, swapping tomato sauce for a broiled red pepper sauce can be similarly delightful, all while giving less potassium per serving.

18. Swiss Chard, Spinach and Beet Greens

Swiss chard, spinach, and beet greens are verdant green vegetables that contain high measures of different supplements and minerals, including potassium.

At the point when served crude, the measure of potassium fluctuates between 140–290 milligrams for every cup. While verdant vegetables therapist to a littler serving size when cooked, the potassium content continues as before.

For instance, a half-cup of crude spinach will psychologist to around 1 tablespoon when cooked. Along these lines, eating a half cup of cooked spinach will contain a lot higher measure of potassium than a half cup of crude spinach.

Moderate utilization of crude Swiss chard, spinach, and beet greens is desirable overcooked greens in order to keep arm's length from high intake of high potassium intake.

19. Dates, Raisins, and Prunes

Dates, raisins and prunes are basic dried organic products. At the point when organic products are dried, the entirety of their supplements are concentrated, including potassium.

For instance, one cup of prunes gives 1,274 milligrams of potassium, which is about multiple times the measure of potassium found in one cup of its crude partner, plums. Besides, only four dates give 668 milligrams of potassium.

Given the striking measure of potassium found in these normal dried organic products, it's ideal to do without while on a renal eating regimen to guarantee potassium levels stay positive.

20. Pretzels, Chips, and Crackers

Ready to-eat nibble nourishments like pretzels, chips, and saltines will, in general, be inadequate in supplements and moderately high in salt.

Additionally, it's anything but difficult to consume much of the suggested bit size of these nourishments, regularly prompting significantly more noteworthy salt admission than planned. Additionally, if chips are produced using potatoes, they will contain a lot of potassium also.

EXTRA TIP

In the event that you have kidney illness, decreasing your potassium, phosphorus, and sodium admission can be a significant part of dealing with the sickness.

The high-sodium, high-potassium, and high-phosphorus nourishments recorded above are likely best constrained or maintained a strategic distance from.

Dietary limitations and supplement admission proposals will change dependent on the seriousness of your kidney harm.

Following a renal eating regimen can appear to be overwhelming and somewhat prohibitive on occasion. In this regard, in order to have a working plan for a renal diet to meet your needs, you have to work closely with your doctor, and renal dietitian.

CHAPTER V: Achieving Weight Loss With Renal Diet

Having plans of weight loss? You may wonder how that will work with your Renal diet. Just like most diets, it is quite tough when one tries to lose weight still flowing in the stream of a renal diet, and thus the results may take a while to become evident. If you eat in a healthy way with the right diet, working with your renal dietitian, and adding physical activities into your routine, you can achieve your weight loss goals and feel healthier.

Why some people on Renal want to lose weight?

If you are overweight or obese and on dialysis, you may benefit from weight loss for the following reasons:
- Better blood sugar control.
- Better blood pressure control.
- Decreased cholesterol and triglyceride levels.
- Increase energy.
- Qualification for a kidney transplant.

Weight-loss guide for individuals on renal diet

There is some useful information that anyone to plan on losing weight must know. At the point when you're on renal Diet, conversing with your dietitian and specialist about changes in your typical eating diet is significant. Your dietitian can assist you with framing just the perfect meal routine that keeps in mind both your renal diet and your desire to get in shape, while your PCP may recommend which exercise is best for you. Share with them what your objectives are so you get exact direction for your weight loss diet.

Weight-loss diet guide for individuals on renal diet

To lose weight, your eating habits and shopping taste would have to be checked, don't skip meals; this often leads to overeating, later on, keep a food journal to record what you eat, refrain from grocery shopping when you're hungry, keep distractions at a minimum while you eat, watch your emotions, and hunger level, avoid nibbling while preparing meals, eat slowly, and before grocery shopping, you should make a list, and ensure stick to it.

Achieving your weight loss goals would be a success if you diligently follow these tips.

Exercise with your doctor's consent

It is advisable to begin your exercise bit by bit, and build up to minimum 30 minutes a day, instead of taking the elevator it's advisable to take the stairs, instead of parking closer to the store, you should park farther away from store entrances, this would give some moments of walking, carry out activities such as swimming, or walking. It should be noted that household chores, such as taking out the trash, gardening, and other everyday activities can be considered exercise, so talk to your PCP about what you do now and what else you may do to get more exercise completed.

Portion size consideration

Portion size may be very deceiving, it is advisable to have a proper sizing of the food until you get a right sense of serving sizes, portions should be the appropriate sizes; see the guidelines below.

- ✓ Fats (butter, salad dressing, etc.)
  1 teaspoon

- ✓ Fruit and vegetables
  Half cup

- ✓ Carbohydrates (grains, starches)
  One full cup

- ✓ Protein (meat, fish, poultry)

3 ounces = size of the palm of your hand

- Use a meal plan, this would help you to determine the right serving serve per day
- When dining out, try not to finish the meal. Take it home instead
- Buy smaller packages. Do this if you have an appetite to eat more than one serving.

Self-Appreciation
The key to achieving this is to set reasonable goals and achieve them, when this is done, reward yourself. Some reward includes going to a movie, take dance lessons, have a bowling night with friends.

Hindrances when carrying out weight-loss routines
Weight loss can be difficult. It takes time and dedication to achieve your weight-loss goals. The difficulties you may face are both physical and emotional. Here are some reasons why Renal Diet patients may be deterred from eating right and exercising.

Physical: Anemia
A few people with interminable kidney sickness who are on dialysis have anemia because of low red platelet count, which causes weariness, brevity of breath, and wooziness. Your primary care physician will build up a treatment plan that will help treat weakness. In the event that you have anemia, request that your primary care physician disclose to you when your blood count is sufficiently high for you to practice securely.

Post-treatment

After in-center dialysis, patients tend to feel powerless afterwards and, in this manner, come up short on the inspiration to work out. Now and then this will keep going for just a short time while others require a decent night's rest. Plan practice after a post-treatment lay or exercise on non-dialysis days.

Peritoneal dialysis (PD)

Individuals on peritoneal dialysis (PD) may experience difficulty getting thinner since they retain glucose (sugar) from the dialysis arrangement. The glucose taken in during dialysis can most times indicate as much as 500 calories for every day. The most ideal approach to stay away from weight gain while on peritoneal dialysis is by utilizing dialysis arrangements with minimal measure of glucose. That implies utilizing progressively 1.5% and 2.5% (yellow) packs and less 4.25% (red) sacks. In the scenario, that this affects your level of liquid, work with your dietitian, and PD medical caretaker to decide the measure of salt and fluids, you ought to eat and drink every day.

Individuals on PD, as a rule, have the opportunity and capacity to exercise, and this ought to be a piece of your everyday schedule. A few people think that it's simpler to practice with an unfilled stomach area as opposed to one loaded up with liquid. This ought to be talked about with your PD medical caretaker and doctor.

Adequate protein

Lessening nourishment intake, for the most part, cuts into the quantity of protein eaten. In the event that great protein intake is insufficient while abstaining from excessive food assumption, they may be a loss on your albumin level and muscle mass. Your dietitian can offer direction to help ensure you eat enough low-fat, top-notch protein. Dietitians can likewise monitor your month to month labs to ensure your albumin isn't dropping.

Emotional: Food choices

Our emotional state sometimes affects our eating habits. Some of the time individuals settle on poor nourishment decisions dependent on their enthusiastic state and gorge when they feel down, miserable, or even glad and need to celebrate.

Keeping the course

Losing weight is not like swinging a magical wand, thus it won't be overnight, without knowing this, you may be tempted to try and make huge changes once which can be sometimes futile. So, it's advisable to set easy to achieve goals and this can turn out to an overall major success.

Having a discussion with your dietitian, regarding the various plans that would properly boost your overall health objectives and way of life, would greatly help. Your dietitian may likewise acquaint you with relevant frozen foods that cut cooking time yet are low in phosphorus and potassium. Ensure to remove pointless calories, for example, high-sugar and high-fat nourishments. If you end up losing weight to be on the transplant list, this shows the health care group that you are so dedicated to your wellbeing.

Give your medicinal services a chance to know that you are attempting to get in shape. Your dry weight should be balanced as you shed pounds, so the right measure of liquid is taken out during every treatment.

SUMMARY

Weight-loss dieting from excessive food intake when you're on dialysis can be an additional test to the dialysis diet. Getting thinner doesn't occur without any forethought and requires a great deal of devotion. Steady changes may assist you with accomplishing better outcomes. The methodology isn't only an adjustment in your eating regimen, yet an adjustment in your way of life. When the objectives that are set are quite reasonable, chat with your medicinal services group about an individualized arrangement, and making great propensities as a major aspect of your daily practice. You may wind up a weight reduction example of overcoming adversity.

CONCLUSION

Every great story must come to an end. Before drawing the closing curtain, I would love to share one last important piece of knowledge with you (Call it the icing on the cake, if you like).

How to be successful in the renal diet program

1. Educate yourself, your family, and your friends about your special renal diet.

This is very important because people around you play a major role in your decision making. Whether you would stick to your diet or get influenced by peers depends more on peers than you. They would need to understand and support your diet, and the close-to-hearts ones can even eat with you occasionally just to ensure you are comfortable.

2. Do you plan to eat out? Then make inquiries.

It is known that restaurants employ various methods to prepare the same dish, whatsoever suites them. So, it is advisable to seek council from someone in charge in order to stay on the safe side of the fence and eat healthy dishes.

3. Find info and encouragement in a CDK support group.

Still, on association, this can't be overemphasized. If everyone in a city begins to eat grapes for breakfast, over time it becomes accepted and normal. So, it is when you get info and support from persons of the same diet. This would help you see and feel more okay with your new renal diet.

4. Focus on the foods you can eat, not the ones you can't.

QUIT complaining and start enjoying. Don't be bothered about what you can't freely eat but rather be ecstatic about the new recipes contained in this renal cookbook and start trying them out.

5. Set up a healthy, organized kitchen. Review the foods you have.

There is always a window to be kind, and this is one of them. Instead of focusing on those things not really healthy for you to eat, why not give it to someone that would appreciate it and be blessed by your generosity. This would go a long way to soothe your heart and make someone else feel better.

6. Improve your health and increase your savings by cooking your own meals.

YES! Cooking is best for a time as this. It helps you plan and save at the same time. Pick a favorite dish from the numerous ones in this cookbook and plan special days for it, then look forward to it. Don't let your eating diet be a boring one.

7. Read food labels carefully to make safe and healthy food choices.

Don't just go about eating whatever you see, as this can greatly affect you. Take a few seconds and go through the label and see whatever may be lurking in that meal and if no alarms are raised, Voila! Have a nice meal.

www.ingramcontent.com/pod-product-compliance
Lightning Source LLC
Chambersburg PA
CBHW060850220526
45466CB00003B/1308